Jan de Vries Guide to Health and Vitality

The Jan de Vries Guide to

Health
and
Vitality

Jan de Vries

MAINSTREAM
PUBLISHING

EDINBURGH AND LONDON

First published in Great Britain in 2006 by
MAINSTREAM PUBLISHING COMPANY
(EDINBURGH) LTD
7 Albany Street
Edinburgh EH1 3UG

ISBN 1 84596 142 0

A catalogue record for this book is available
from the British Library

Typeset in Garamond and Helvetica
Printed and bound in Great Britain by
William Clowes Ltd, Beccles, Suffolk

Contents

Energy – Source of Life

Some time ago, as I walked in the Swiss Alps with Alfred Vogel, we both admired the beauty of nature. We talked about the energy in plants, roots, trees and flowers, and the energy of man. We both thought that it is difficult to understand energy or to give an accurate definition of life, and we concluded that we probably only scratch the surface. In actual fact, we knew very little of life energy until the nineteenth century. Nowadays, we know a bit more, namely that life is a constant renewal of cell tissues and cells. Looking around, Vogel remarked how wonderful life was and how rewarding it was to live in that breathtaking country of Switzerland, to see energy radiating to the surroundings from the sun. Being high up in the mountains, we were that much closer to it.

While walking, we also discussed the many problems that are apparent in the world today. Why are so many people ill? Why are there such widespread, global diseases? Life expectancy might be longer nowadays, hygiene has improved, and we have a better control over most illnesses and diseases, but why is the quality of life often so poor? Why are we faced with an enormous increase in cases of cancer and degenerative diseases? Is it purely because people are living longer, or are there other reasons? As we pondered these issues, I remarked what a pity it was that disasters such as the Chernobyl accident as well as other negative atmospheric influences were affecting the whole world, even there in the beauty of the Swiss Alps.

Do we understand energy as a source of life? What are we really doing with it and what is our part in this great field of energy? As Vogel and I admired the power and life energy of even the smallest flower or herb that grew in the Swiss Alps, we were aware that the same life force also exists in man, and that this can easily be disturbed or influenced, either positively or negatively. It is therefore crucial that the life force or vital force produces the right type of energy and is dealt with properly.

It is essential that we learn how to deal with this vital force, which is given to all that grows, for throughout our lives it is faced with threats and obstacles. Look, for example, at the miracle of the birth of a baby. When a baby is born, it gets the breath of life, the energy by which it will live, and then what happens to it? It is faced with all kinds of interferences. A breastfed baby is extremely lucky, but very often a child is either fed with cow's-milk products or adulterated food which does not give it the right vital force for life. Pure mother's milk gives a baby the best possible start in life – a very good vital force. However, this lessens when the child is fed on a milk product, which usually contains much higher levels of proteins than mother's milk; but still the baby manages to grow. Then the infant, with its vital force, is faced with interference in the form of immunisation. Although this is perhaps necessary nowadays, it is nevertheless a huge attack on the baby's immune system.

As the infant develops and starts school, it will be influenced by all the viral and bacterial activities surrounding it, with the result that its immune system is faced with another shock and needs to be built up. The child does not always eat food which has life in it, such as fresh fruit and vegetables, which is important to boost the necessary reserves as it grows up. Energy is very important and the child's energy is very much influenced by what it eats. Does it get enough sleep? Does it get the right food to eat? Does it get enough rest? Good health depends on the sources of the body's energy and whether the body is getting what it needs.

As the child becomes an adult, it continues to need the right food and the right nutrition to perform what is necessary for daily life. A job can sometimes be extremely taxing and if someone finds work exhausting or stressful, the first signs of degeneration can become apparent. Every day, I hear people saying how difficult it is for them to cope with life or that even on awakening they feel tired. After a good night's sleep and with the right nourishment, we should be able to cope with life and work. As I have said, this is a time when degeneration can start – sometimes even before we reach the age of 40. We therefore need to ensure that we have a good balance in our food pattern between acidity, alkalinity, proteins and carbohydrates. This is very important, as we shall discover later in this book. We often see that, with all the stresses of life, if a person suffers from poor nutrition as well, there is invariably a breakdown of the cell tissue.

Then, as we get older, we come across people with a form of senility, Alzheimer's disease, which brings about forgetfulness. It is so sad to see the effects of this cruel disease on intelligent people, those we have known in the sporting, acting or scientific worlds. What can be done about it? It is very important that we eat the right foods and that we look at our lifestyle, so that we can reach a ripe old age and still enjoy life to the full. I always think of my older patients, some over 100 years old, who are still determined to live as healthily as they can. They eat the right foods to keep their arteries clear and take remedies to keep their circulation in good working order and their minds fresh.

I remember Vogel and I were once walking in Korea when we came across an elderly man picking one ginkgo leaf after another. I said to Vogel, 'Does he not realise that he is taking an overdose?' Vogel suggested that I talk to him. Fortunately, he spoke English, and when I asked him why he took so many ginkgo leaves, he replied that he took them every day and had done so for a very long time. Ginkgo is known as 'the memory tree', and he wanted to keep his mind alert. I then commented that he was taking this remedy in overdose quantities, to which he replied that he was well over 100 years of age and it had never done him any harm! He made certain that what he put in his body not only kept his blood circulation healthy but also kept his mind sharp. We cannot go through life thinking we have a problem and that we just have to live with it. It is the quality of life that is important and I am encouraged when I look around at people who in old age enjoy health, happiness and vitality. We should all follow their example and respect the life that is given to us.

Over the years, I have worked with people who have known a lot about energy. I have also seen how people have used energy and have taught others what they can do with it. In my book *Body Energy*, I suggested many guidelines on what one can do oneself in order to balance energy and how we can positively influence the vital force which is in every one of us. During the many years I have been in practice, I have seen people who felt they had come to the end of the road and who thought 'this is it'. It was not until I could unlock their minds and advise them on how much they could influence their energy with some very simple techniques that they realised this was not so. Sometimes this changed their lives and brought about the necessary relief to enable them to carry on and enjoy life for another 20 or 30 years.

We have to learn how to work with and how to balance energy.

Balancing energy is very important. For instance, the centre of gravity should be in the correct position and it is for that reason that I often find it crucial to carry out spinal manipulation and spinal corrections. We often see when people have simple neck or back problems, where there is either an imbalance to the left or the right, that their bodies can be likened to a ship that capsizes when it is overladen on one side instead of being equally balanced on all sides, or to a watch in which the smallest wheel doesn't turn properly, thus stopping it from ticking. The body can often be like this, when the centre of gravity is out of balance and health deteriorates, and yet this can so easily be put right. If there is an imbalance in one's health, then there are reasons for this and we must do everything possible to restore that balance.

In my practice, I often see patients in whom the balance of energy is wrong. When I ask myself where the energy is disturbed in a patient, I sometimes have to take on the role of detective to find out. Once this has been established, there is so much that one can do. A young lady came to see me some time ago. When she walked into my consulting room, I could see that she was walking very much to one side. I discovered that her jaw was out of place. After I adjusted her jaw, I could see almost in minutes that she started to straighten up. Her body was, as I say, like an unbalanced ship on the sea. It is very important to make sure that energy in the body has freedom to move around. On another, more recent occasion, a gentleman consulted me and I saw that he was having problems with his body gravity. With the help of copper and zinc magnets, I managed to balance him, and he was so much happier.

I enjoyed the time I spent studying in China, where I learned some valuable techniques to correct imbalances between left and right, positive and negative. When observing a patient, I think of what I was taught there – to *look*, to *listen* and to *feel*, to discover where the energy balance is disturbed or where the endocrine system might be disordered, listening to the tone of the patient's voice, feeling the temperature of the body, taking the pulse or examining the tongue. By doing this, I can decide what needs to be done to harmonise the body. Even minor problems can disturb the body's balance and hinder it from working efficiently.

I would like to share with my readers some of the ideas that Dr Leonard Allan and I have studied and developed. On the surface, they might seem complicated, but they can bring about such tremendous benefits. Let's have a look at who and what we really are, and what can be done to influence the body's energy.

ENERGY IS THE WHOLE HUMAN BEING

If you look at the diagram on the facing page, which Dr Allan and I created, you will see that the basic part of a human being is 'I am'. This 'I am' means that every person is endowed with the faculties of a mind, a body, a soul and a heart. These faculties allow us physical, mental, emotional and spiritual lives, which we express by looking around and observing, thinking, feeling and acting. The way in which these faculties function therefore affects our appearance and attitude, our abilities and the way we communicate – in other words, the self that we present to the world.

The diagram works in two ways. If we start from the outer layer, we know that naturopaths look at a patient's appearance to help them determine what the inner problem is with that person's health. On the other hand, working from the inside out, the diagram illustrates that our mind influences our mental state, which then in turn affects our thought processes and thus our ability to function effectively. A clear example of this would be when a person's lack of self-belief inhibits them from completing a task. If, however, a human being is able to think positively, this will help them to achieve the result they are aiming for.

The point is not only that the aspects of life arranged on each side of the square affect one another. The sides of the square are not separated – every element of our being is connected with all the others. Endeavour to understand this diagram and you will understand yourself and others. You will be able to detect an area of deficiency or an imbalance in mind, body, soul and heart.

The diagram also shows us the futility of merely treating the symptoms of an imbalance in the body. Only by discovering the real cause of the symptom and addressing that can we achieve true health.

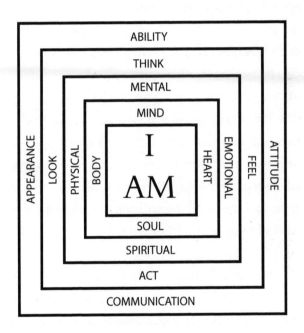

Understanding the whole human being

Throughout the universe, fatigue is the main thing that leads to distortion and destruction. The human body is no exception to this rule. Where there is fatigue, the joints become strained and skeletal relationships are changed; muscles operating around such joints are stretched. One must remember that it is gravity that underlies it all. The four essentials underlying the preservation of life are proper food, proper temperature, proper rest, proper elimination. All these factors depend on gravity in the last analysis.

A perfectly balanced body can stand with feet together, eyes closed and muscles relaxed. The bones support the weight of the body and are not subject to fatigue. Any distortion of the body structure changes the balance, so the bones are no longer in a position to support the weight of the body and the muscles must contract to hold the body upright. Thus the muscles become subject to fatigue.

The intelligent use of methods of applying the hands to certain areas of the body helps to eliminate fatigue and thus produce a balance of the body energies. Such a treatment will relax the tissues and take the load off the body and mind. The body feels as light as a feather and all work and movement is done without effort. In this restored condition, all the energy that was required merely to exist is freed and turned into productivity and progress. It is very important that cellular and intercellular tensions are corrected so as to remove all strain – in short, to bring all matter back to maximum usefulness by the correction of fatigue.

Warning Signs

Thousands of years ago, the Ancient Chinese found that the abdominal area had reflex zones which refer to certain areas of the body or organs. Pain in these zones indicates a developing state of disease – a sort of warning of things to come. The next diagram plots these abdominal areas. The abbreviations denote the organ that could be in trouble if pain develops.

The ancients have left many gems of wisdom for us to apply. The age-old saying is 'Look, Listen, Feel'. With this in mind, here are some indicators which can help you to monitor your body's condition and look out for potential problems.

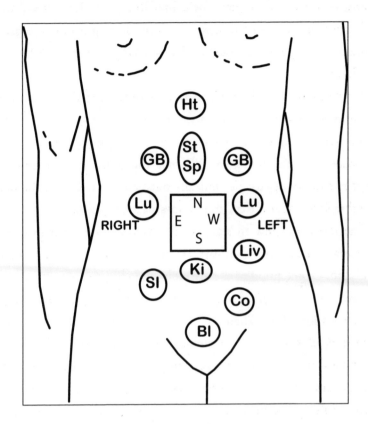

The abdominal reflex zones

Key: Ht = heart; GB = gall bladder; St = stomach; Sp = spleen; Lu = lung; Ki = kidneys; Liv = liver; SI = small intestine; Co = colon; Bl = bladder

The eyes

When we grow old, the white of our eyes shows between the iris and the bottom eyelid. A younger adult with the white showing is in a very negative condition. The organs are weakened, and the person in question will have poor reflexes in case of danger and hence be prone to accidents. A prominent red colour in the whites of the eyes is a sign of a bad liver. The liver has grown tired, perhaps due to an over-consumption of food, especially animal products. When the red has spread all over the whites of the eyes, the organs are malfunctioning. A white ring around the iris indicates malfunctioning in the abdominal area. Bulging eyes indicate thyroid trouble. Large, very convex eyes denote a well-developed muscular system.

Frequent blinking can signify that the body is attempting to discharge excess negative energy in any way it can. One should not blink one's eyes more than three times per minute. If the eyes move constantly or are slow to react (to follow your finger, for example), there is a problem with the heart – the pace of the heart is not normal. In such cases, the pupil of the eye will be too big.

Swelling around the eyes, particularly swelling of the upper eyelid, indicates gallstones. When the stones pass, the swelling will drop immediately. A dark brown colour under the eyes indicates excessive positive kidneys and trouble in the female organs. Swelling under the eyes indicates kidney stones, gallstones or blood stagnation. Dark blue or violet shadows under the eyes reveal blood stagnation, probably caused by an over-consumption of fruit, sugar and meat.

Pimples on the interior of the eyelid signify excess protein. They usually appear and disappear relatively quickly. If the inside of the eyelid is almost white, this signifies anaemia. It should be red. To examine, gently pinch the eyelid and pull it away from the eye.

A broad thick eyebrow is positive. A thin eyebrow is negative. Too much sweet food, especially sugar, makes the eyebrows thinner and eventually causes them to disappear. People with almost no eyebrows are prone to cancer.

The nose

An examination of the nose can tell much about the condition of the body. Reduce your intake of food and you will see your nose grow smaller. A long nose starting high up on the face is negative. A short nose indicates a strong constitution. A small nose pointing upwards is a sign of strong, positive energy. If the bridge of the nose is broad and high, this normally indicates a healthy, effectively functioning stomach.

The nose indicates the condition of the heart. An enlarged nose shows an enlarged heart as a result of excess eating and drinking. A fat nose that is somewhat oily and sometimes shiny indicates over-consumption of animal protein. Red blood vessels on the tip of the nose are an indication of high blood pressure and a sign that heart disease will follow.

The nostrils show the condition of the lungs – the larger the nostrils, the better. Small nostrils indicate weak lungs.

The mouth

A small mouth is positive. A large mouth is negative. A horizontal line between the mouth and nose shows a malfunctioning of the sexual organs. The lips should be of equal thickness. In general, thick lips indicate a positive constitution and thin lips a negative constitution. Dry, thin lips are a sign of underactivity of the glands. The size of the upper lip shows the condition of the liver. If the lip is swollen, the liver is enlarged. This may also suggest that the subject eats too much or is prone to mental disorders. The size of the lower lip indicates the condition of the large intestine. When the lower lip is swollen, there is a weakness, a looseness, in the intestines, and thus constipation. Epilepsy is a possibility when both lips are enlarged. This may also indicate that the person in question was given too much food as a child. If a woman's lips are straight, with no downward curve, she may have problems with breastfeeding. The length of the upper lip denotes the strength of the spine. A short upper lip is a sign of a weak spinal column.

The lips should usually be pink. However, they grow darker with age. A young person with dark lips has poor circulation, perhaps due to an excessive intake of animal protein and strong foods. People with dark lips tend to develop cancer, pineal troubles and diseases of the sexual organs. If the centre of the upper lip is full, red and moist, this denotes a strong, healthy reproductive system.

The texture of the lips reveals the condition of the stomach. A cyst on the right side of the mouth indicates stomach trouble, acidity or the beginning of an ulcer in the left side of the stomach. A cyst on the left side of the mouth indicates a problem in the right side of the stomach.

Some other facial reflex zones

- A wide chin denotes strong kidneys. A narrow, pointed chin denotes a tendency to develop kidney disease.
- Pale cheeks with red spots show intestinal disorders. Extreme paleness of the cheeks means intestinal inactivity.
- A broad, high forehead, fine skin and hair, bright eyes and ears positioned well forward denote a well-developed nervous system and brain.
- The longer the septum, the better the liver is developed and the more able it is to fulfil its work. A short septum signifies the reverse.

As we can see from the above, the health problems we are faced with in the stressful, polluted world today are many. In the chapters that follow I will show you how to improve your overall health and get the most out of your body.

In order to understand how body energy works and the disciplines that one can adopt to influence the vital force, we have to consider a few things. How do we regain energy when we are tired every day or wake up in the morning feeling tired? What can we do about this? First, we have to look at three sources of our energy – food, water and air. We can control the foods we eat and the water we drink. We can choose to eat a synthetic pudding or a tin of tomato soup that has never seen a tomato if we prefer, or we can choose foods which have life in them – organic foods, for example. However, the air we breathe is largely out of our control. The air we breathe in will, in all probability, be polluted. The effects of pollution are apparent in the tremendous increase in degenerative diseases.

If we get enough energy from our food and water and we have a good immune system, our bodies can cope with pollution in the air. It is therefore important that we have good dietary management and that we carefully examine what we eat. The majority of people do not realise that the body needs 91 nutrients. It may only take a deficiency in one or two vitamins, minerals or trace elements for us to become ill. If we drink a lot of artificial liquids containing additives, preservatives and so on, we can become really ill; or if we consume foods containing the wrong ingredients, this can start off a degenerative disease. We must realise that we will only get out of life what we put into it. That is a very important message.

We also need rest, relaxation and exercise for good body energy. It is essential that we walk, swim, cycle or undertake some sporting activity or exercise that will restore energy and not damage it. We therefore need the right type of exercise and restful sleep, which will be discussed later in the book. In addition to relaxation, we may sometimes benefit from taking suitable natural remedies to restore energy that has been disturbed by either disease or imbalance. Of course, we need fresh air and plenty of it. This is especially so if you work in a busy office where you are exposed to fluorescent lights and computer screens, both of which attack our vital energy.

We must bear in mind that we belong to nature, we are born in nature and we have to work with nature in order to live life to the full with plenty of health and vitality.

CHAPTER ONE

A Healthy Digestive System

This chapter is one of the most important in this book. Over the years I have been involved in broadcasting, as well as writing articles for newspapers and magazines, I have found that the majority of questions I am asked relate to the digestive system. Some time ago, I was interviewed by Gloria Hunniford on Radio 2. I remember discussing digestion and the problems associated with irritable bowel syndrome (IBS). Following this programme, I received an astonishing 8,400 letters from listeners who wanted more information.

The digestive system is very closely linked to the energy we have – or produce – in our lifetime. There are a great number of influences that can interfere with the digestive system and, even more importantly, the absorption of our food, and a lot of problems are self-induced. As I said in the introduction, we need 91 nutrients to live. Each of these is significant and if we omit even one or two, then complications can occur. When we look at our diet, first of all we need to ask ourselves what kind of food we are eating, whether there is any life in it and, if so, have we killed that life? For instance, in steaming vegetables, we retain 90 per cent of their nutrients. If we boil them, this reduces to 60 per cent or sometimes less and if we microwave them, there is only 5 per cent of the original nutritional value remaining in them. If we consume adulterated food containing additives and colourings, the digestive system repeatedly gets a big knock. If we combine the wrong food pattern with doses of stress, this can lead to IBS. We do not need to look very far to understand why this occurs and how closely it is linked to depletion of energy.

The other day, I was sitting across from an interesting gentleman who was interviewing me for a radio programme. While we were talking, he had to excuse himself several times to relieve himself of wind, whereupon he confided in me that he was greatly troubled with IBS. I remarked that in the short time I had been with him he had drunk three cups of coffee. So I asked him how many he drank each day. Believe it or not, he told me he drank 18 mugfuls! Coffee is, in fact, one of the main contributors to IBS. This poor man, not only having to cope with the stressful job of being a radio presenter but also filling himself with coffee (containing sugar and milk), was asking for trouble. This was simply a case of drinking and eating the wrong foods, which, coupled with high doses of stress, resulted in IBS.

Some sufferers may think, 'Well, it is only IBS,' and many doctors often say you just have to live with it, but IBS can lead to many problems, as I have seen repeatedly. Never underestimate a problem and never disregard an alarm bell. To reiterate what I have said in many of my books and also during lectures, you cannot ignore an alarm bell. If the church is on fire and the bells are ringing, it is very easy to stop the bells ringing, but if you don't get the water hose out, then the fire will rage on and the destruction will get worse and worse. It is the same when we have a headache or IBS. It is easy to take an aspirin, an antacid or whatever to stop the bells ringing, as it were, but the symptoms will not improve unless the underlying problem is investigated.

In studying the way in which people eat, I have noticed that they do not allow their bodies sufficient time to properly digest their food. Once, when I was in the States, I was followed by a man who called himself 'the Juice Man'. At every lecture I gave, he spoke to members of my audience, telling them that Jan de Vries believed in fresh fruit and fresh vegetable juices and that, as he was 'the Juice Man' he could help them. Although what he did was thoughtful, I didn't agree. I always tell people that God has given us teeth to chew and, by chewing, we get the correct saliva needed to break down our foods, which is the best digestive aid there is. Many people eat their food as quickly as possible, but this will only cause problems.

I clearly remember the time when Alfred Vogel and I reached the decision to create what is now known as the *Detox Box*. While we were having a meal in a hotel, an attractive-looking family came in. I was puzzled as to why they all had round, chubby faces, and I mentioned my concern to Vogel. I knew there must be something wrong with them. I soon realised what it was when their food was placed before them. They didn't take any time to taste what they were eating but just gobbled it down. In no time at all, they had finished their meal and left. It was then that I remarked to Vogel that their food could be doing them nothing but harm. It was eaten so quickly that they had not given it time to be digested or absorbed by their bodies. It was that particular incident that prompted us to devise the *Detox Box,* which now, years later, continues to go from strength to strength. It is a natural, easy-to-use ten-day elimination programme. It comprises four preparations from Bioforce: *Calendula Complex, Frangula Complex, Milk Thistle Complex* and *Solidago Complex.* In actual fact, I use this myself every spring and autumn to give my body a thorough but gentle clean, which can be likened to someone thoroughly cleaning their house. Not only does it purify the stomach, the lungs, the gall bladder, the liver and the kidneys but it also aids the elimination of toxins from the entire system and is extremely beneficial in maintaining health and harmony in the body.

As good digestion is essential, I feel it is necessary that attention be paid to this matter. I have therefore decided to revisit some of the views expressed in one of my earlier books, *Ten Golden Rules for Good Health*. Because they look at digestion as a whole, which is vital, I thought it would be a good idea to recap on these ten golden rules.

The ten rules for healthy eating are of paramount importance when one is striving for good health. There are many diseases that are caused by a poor diet and an unhealthy lifestyle. Now you probably wish to know what you should change in order to successfully prevent these problems or perhaps to undo any harm which has already been done.

Many diseases and health problems – I hardly have to stress – are not destiny, but the results of our way of living. There are things in life which one cannot, or can only with difficulty, change, such as the condition of our environment. But other things can be quite easily influenced. One of these is our nutrition. If you deal consciously and intelligently with the problem of your eating habits, it will pay dividends many times over. Nutrition not only determines the state of our digestive systems but also influences in an indirect manner, by way of our blood and lymphatic fluids, all the other organs in our bodies.

Now, what would we call 'a healthy way of eating'? After looking at the historical background of our development and at our biology, the answer is easy: healthy food is that which the human being, in the course of its evolution, has found in its natural environment. The body has adapted to this kind of food and it is easily digestible. Modern nutrition in the industrial countries hardly fulfils these requirements. A short-term adjustment of the body to society's new nutritional conditions has been impossible, and the consequences are logical and in accordance with this. If humanity had been able, one million years ago, to eat as we eat today, an adequate adaptation might have been possible. The intestines would have become shorter, the pancreas and the liver would have become bigger and the teeth and the lower jaw would have become smaller.

Now, in order to eat healthily, we should follow as much as possible the example of our ancestors. We should try to eat the food which, over the long stretch of human history, has become natural to us. As our 'normal' nutrition, today's way of eating, is much different from the ancient way of eating, the following rules may seem very demanding to you at first. However, this does not mean going without food that you like altogether. Food should and has to taste good! Even when following these ten rules exactly, you can have meals which are in no way inferior to 'nouvelle cuisine'. If your body were able to talk to you, it would probably advise you to follow these ten rules for healthy nutrition, which would assist you in having a long and healthy life.

TEN RULES FOR HEALTHY LIVING

1. The main part of the diet should be of plant origin. Fruit, vegetables and salads should, with grain products and potatoes, be the basis of nutrition. These foods should take up at least 70 per cent of the entire intake. In this way, a high fibre content is guaranteed, which is absolutely essential for the digestion.

2. Raw, uncooked food should not be the exception but an important part of your daily nutrition. When half of our food is of plant origin and is eaten raw, this is excellent for our health. When there is no inflammation of the intestines, more of this kind of food can be eaten.

3. Meat, poultry and fish should, as a general rule, be eaten only once a week. One can give these up for long periods without problems.

4. The proportion of fat in food should not be more than 20–30 per

cent. Animal fat should be avoided as much as possible. Instead, plant fats (unsaturated oils) should be used.

5. The more natural the food is (this means not industrially prefabricated), the better it is.

6. You should live completely, or almost completely, without sugar. As a guideline, you should use no more sugar than salt.

7. There should be long intervals between meals. General rule: five hours. Longer intervals will never harm you.

8. Sour milk products are much better than regular milk products.

9. Drink plenty. Water or herb teas are ideal. Fizzy drinks should be avoided.

10. Alcohol should only be drunk in small quantities.

NORMAL AND ABNORMAL DIGESTION

The digestive organs and teeth of human beings suggest that they belong in the category of fructivores (fruit eaters). This does not mean that humans should live exclusively on fruit, but it does show that, by nature, they are best suited to eating cereals, roots, fruit, nuts and many other products of the soil. This does not exclude them from eating animal produce once in a while. However, one must understand that animal protein is basically a 'second-hand' food, as most of the energy an animal receives from plant food has already been used by its own body.

Only about 20 per cent of our modern food remains natural. We eat far too much animal protein, refined carbohydrates and the wrong kind of fat. We eat too much, too fast, too often and usually at the wrong time of the day.

Unsuitable nutrition is one of the major causes of our civilisation's diseases and of our disastrous state of health. The second cause is the wrong kind of medical treatment.

Digestion in the Mouth

The normal process

As food in former times was hard, rough, tough and fibrous, people had to chew it thoroughly for a long time. All carbohydrates from bread, cereals, potatoes, rice, etc. were broken up by enzymes in the saliva and thus prepared for digestion in the stomach and the intestines. The food was mixed with up to 1.5 litres of saliva each day, and specific antibodies in the mouth ensured that innumerable bacteria and toxins were destroyed there. The chewing also stimulated the blood circulation of the gums and dental decay was rare.

The abnormal process

As our modern food is soft and contains very little fibre, we no longer have to chew so thoroughly. Many things are swallowed before being saturated with saliva and thus some of the carbohydrates in the food cannot be broken up. Every year, more additives and other artificial substances find their way into food, and the antibodies in the mouth are unable to detoxify such quantities.

Many toxins then pass into the throat, where the defence mechanism of the tonsils cannot always cope with so much work. They become enlarged and inflamed, causing difficulty in breathing. Today, we see many children with their mouths agape, not due to lack of intelligence, but mainly because the defence mechanism of their lymphatic systems, which includes the tonsils, is continually overstrained through an over-consumption of dairy produce, sweets and soft drinks. In earlier days, the tonsils were often removed when they became inflamed, but the medical fraternity has now learned that they fulfil important tasks in the human body and that their removal provides only temporary help. The cause of swelling and inflammation is not eliminated, and the side effects, such as bronchitis, asthma and sinus problems, still remain. The only remedy lies in an immediate change of diet and intensive natural treatment.

As people no longer chew properly, dentists only rarely see gums which receive a healthy blood supply. The roots of the teeth are undernourished and gradually become loose. When the body lacks certain minerals and other nutrients, its most important task is to make sure that the essential organs receive all the vital nutrients available. The survival of the entire organism depends upon this. The health of teeth and bones is a lower priority for the body, and therefore in an emergency the required minerals are removed from the easily dissolved mineral deposits of the bones and teeth. Thus one can understand that tooth decay is not only a local problem but also a sign of a general, complicated disturbance of the entire organism. Not only elderly people but even babies and small children can suffer from a lack of minerals and from a degeneration of the jawbone.

As a result of modern malnutrition, the composition of the saliva changes and bacteria thrive through constant contact with sugar and sweets. The waste products of these bacteria in the mouth cause hyperacidity and this acid attacks the dental enamel. Most of our modern food is far too acidic and, in the long run, all of these different kinds of acid will destroy our teeth. Not only things that taste acidic but also any kind of sugar or sweets provoke an acid reaction in our digestive tracts.

You can prove to yourself quite easily that acids can destroy your teeth. In order to do a test, put some vinegar or lemon juice into a little jar and then place a small bone or a tooth in the jar and screw on the lid. If after some weeks you open the jar again, you will find that the little bone or the tooth is not there any more: it will have been dissolved by the acid. So please beware of acids and sweets!

Factors like malnutrition, acidity and bacteria interact, and caries (decay), tartar and pyorrhoea develop. These problems cannot be prevented, even by intensive brushing of the teeth, particularly as the consumption of sugar and sweets increases each year. But, after all, the food industry should be allowed to do business! Sooner or later, the teeth begin to fall out and people need dentures. Already 90 per cent of all school-age children have caries.

Albert von Haller proved many years ago in *Gefährdete Menschheit* (*Endangered Humanity*) that primitive people who start eating white flour, sugar and sweets will, within a few years, show symptoms of nutritional deficiency, beginning with tooth decay.

Digestion in the Stomach

The normal process

Food is liquidised in the mouth, thereby breaking up all the carbohydrates into different parts, which then pass through the gullet (oesophagus) into the stomach, where the nutrient solution is kneaded for a long time with the acidic gastric juices by the contractions of the stomach wall. At the same time, the transformation of starches into sugar takes place, special enzymes digest all the proteins from the food and the stomach acid kills the remaining harmful bacteria and neutralises toxic substances.

The stomach wall is covered by a layer of mucus, which is renewed constantly and therefore cannot be attacked by the gastric acid. Depending on the kind of food, the nutrient solution remains between one and eight hours in the stomach. When its work is completed, the stomach slowly empties its contents into the upper part of the small intestines, namely the duodenum.

The abnormal process

When the nutrients have not been sufficiently liquidised in the mouth, the carbohydrates cannot be fully broken up. These nutrients then enter the stomach, where a more intensive digestion is needed. The nutrient solution may contain many indigestible substances, such as sugar, white flour and fruit juices. For such foods, there are no adequate digestive juices available. Glands which could produce such juices would have to be developed first. For this reason, it may still be a very long time before human beings are able to digest such refined foods without problems.

Nevertheless, the stomach does make an effort to digest these concentrates and provides huge quantities of normal digestive juices for this alien food. As only very little of these juices will actually be used, the rest remain in the stomach, with the risk that these very acidic juices will irritate and eventually destroy part of the stomach wall. In order to prevent this, the organism will begin to produce vast quantities of mucus. However, a stomach filled with mucus cannot digest food properly, and the nutrient solution stays for far too long in the stomach, where it begins to ferment and produces much gas. People suffer from wind and a tight feeling in their abdomen. Sometimes, if animal protein and starches are eaten at the same time, the transformation of starches cannot take place because of the high degree of acidity. Of course, this depends on the different quantities of animal protein and starches eaten during a meal. Because of this, many of my patients follow the advice given in *Fit for Life* by Marilyn and Harvey Diamond, and similar health books, and try not to eat starches and animal protein at the same meal.

Digestion in the Small Intestine
The normal process
When the nutrient solution leaves the stomach, it is slowly passed on into the duodenum, where it is mixed with the juices secreted by the pancreas and the gall bladder. The bile from the gall bladder breaks up fats, which are then transported via the lymph glands to the liver. The juices of the pancreas are alkaline and neutralise the nutrient solution after it has left the very acidic milieu of the stomach. The nutrient solution is then pushed further into the small intestine, where the digestion becomes more intensive.

The intestines are moving constantly in order to mix the nutrient solution with the gastric juices. About five hours later, the digestion in the small intestine has been completed. Gradually, the various food components are assimilated via small filters located in the wall of the intestines. The nutrients are then passed into a net of tiny blood vessels (capillaries) located in and behind the intestinal wall. The filtered blood from all these tiny vessels then flows into a much larger blood vessel (the vena porta) and from there it goes into the liver, where it is cleansed once again.

The abnormal process

The partly digested nutrient solution is slowly pushed from the stomach into the duodenum. However, when gas pressure builds up because of huge quantities of mucus, the entire stomach contents may suddenly be emptied into the duodenum. When this happens, the digestive juices of the intestines cannot neutralise all the acid in the nutrient solution quickly enough and the acid then attacks the intestinal wall. Thus inflammation or even ulcers can develop.

Nowadays, I see in my daily practice more and more people suffering from gastric and intestinal diseases. Most people do not realise that such diseases could easily have been prevented, and that is a great pity. The body's production of key substances such as hormones and proteins is dependent on the food we eat and its effective digestion and hence absorption into our blood through the filters in the intestinal wall.

Digestion in the Large Intestine

The normal process

After all the nutrients are assimilated into the blood, the fibre and other residual substances of the nutrient solution pass into the large intestine. There, billions of bacteria accomplish important tasks. They live on the fibre, from which they extract the last of the nutrients. These bacteria are very important to us: they produce vitamins, especially those of the B group, and help to eliminate harmful substances and germs. They have many more functions about which we still know very little.

Also in the large intestine, the nutrient solution is pushed further down by the movements of the ring muscles of the intestinal wall. The more fibre there is, the more the nerves in the intestinal wall will be stimulated and the sooner the excrement, by way of the bowels, can be disposed of. Sometimes, this process can be influenced by psychological problems but, on the whole, the composition of the daily food is the most important factor in preventing hard excrement.

The nutrient solution, which is very liquid in the small intestine, loses more and more fluid during its passage through the large intestine. The further the nutrient solution travels into the lower sections of the bowels, the more compact it becomes. Fibrous substances play an important part here. They are able to retain a lot of water and they see to it that the excrement does not become too dry. Good excrement is still about 70 per cent water and is not sticky.

Dr Denis Burkitt, an Irish physician and scientist, world famous for his books and publications on the value of fibre in our food, examined the eating habits of African tribes in the year 1971. He compared these with the eating habits of Europeans and discovered that the tribes ate much fibrous food, which passed through their intestines in less than 30 hours, the weight of the excrement being between 300 and 500 g. A European's excrement weighed between 80 and 120 g and the average time it took to pass through the intestines was 70 hours. Burkitt believed that many of our Western diseases, from which the Africans suffer only exceptionally, are caused mainly by a lack of fibre in the diet.

The excrement of a healthy person contains only a small quantity of food at the end of its journey through the large intestine and the colon, or even no food at all. It contains mainly bacteria, skin flakes and useless substances.

The abnormal process

If we always ate food which was appropriate to our digestive systems, we would – as you have seen – digest everything without any problem. When, however, we eat food which is unsuitable for our organism, exactly the opposite happens. Day by day, we make so many nutritional errors that it is hard to say which is the worst. Doubtless, a combination of different mistakes continually made is the most important cause of our so-called 'civilisation diseases'.

While describing abnormal digestive processes, I mentioned how, through a sudden gas pressure, the nutrient solution can get into the lower sections of the intestines. The upper part of the small intestine is practically sterile, but further down there are innumerable bacteria that live exclusively on fibre and food residues. These different strains of bacteria are very useful to us and they normally remain in balance, meaning that none of them can multiply in such a way as to be dangerous to our health. When, however, there is suddenly an abundance of undigested food, this balance is disturbed in favour of harmful bacteria, which then have a real feast. These 'putrefactive' bacteria multiply very fast, and their metabolic waste (excrement) causes the formation of gas and dangerous toxins, like indole and scatole. The person in question feels bloated and gets stomachache, and the abdomen swells.

The immune system of the large intestine is thus continually overstrained, and alien substances, toxins and/or harmful bacteria enter the body tissues. As a result of the irritant effect of these substances, there is the possibility of inflammation of any part of the body. A typical example is ulcers of the anus, which are more commonplace than one would think possible in our time. Another problem is ever-increasing fungal disease. Fungi can only multiply unchecked when most of the enteric (gut-friendly) bacteria have been destroyed by antibiotics, or in some other way. The consumption of refined carbohydrates supports the growth of fungi, as they prefer to live on sugar, like many other small creatures. A fungal infection can spread to any part of the body and cause dangerous diseases. More and more people are dying from fungal infections.

WHAT ABOUT SNACKS BETWEEN MEALS?

Not long ago, doctors used to think that it was healthier to eat small quantities of food several times during the day instead of large meals and that this would make the digestion of food easier. This idea is not altogether wrong, as nobody should eat too much food at one time. However, it has now been proved that, even for diabetics, eating between meals is wrong, as a general rule, as the following happens.

As soon as the nutrient solution reaches the stomach, digestion begins. This process, depending upon the kind of food eaten, takes an average of four to five hours. After this food has been digested in the stomach, it will slowly be passed into the duodenum. If, at such a moment, new, undigested food comes into the stomach, it will be passed directly into the upper intestines together with the already digested food and will be the cause of many health problems. Only the already digested nutrients can pass through the very small filters of the intestinal wall. The rest stays in the small intestine much too long and begins to ferment.

Although a certain amount of fermentation is completely normal, semi-digested food causing super-fermentation in the upper part of the small intestine can then, because of air pressure, be pushed into the large intestine or even lower. This can cause much gas, pain and inflammation. It is therefore better not to eat between meals, except perhaps some fruit once in a while, which will be quickly digested.

It is the task of the small intestine to break up the food into its basic substances, such as carbohydrates, proteins, fats, vitamins, minerals, etc. Because of our modern eating habits, this task has become very difficult. The nutrient solution often contains molecules which can only be digested with much effort, and there is usually a high concentration of unnatural substances.

In the long run, the residual toxins and irritating substances damage the sensitive intestinal wall, and the small filters which it contains become either clogged or porous. In this way, more and more useless substances end up in the capillaries or in the surrounding tissues. The rest of the nutrient solution (undigested food, fibre, chemicals and other unnatural substances) is now pushed into the bowels by alternating contraction and relaxation of the ring muscles of the bowels.

BOTTLENECKS IN THE INTESTINES

The muscular movements of the intestines are controlled by hormones and triggered off by neural impulses. If, however, the food contains too little fibre, the network of nerves in the intestinal wall will not be sufficiently stimulated, the bowel movements slow down and the continuous supply of food causes blockages in the intestinal loops (bends). The food residue remains too long in these bends; it ferments, turns bad, becomes dry and hardens. In these areas, inflammation can easily develop. It may take years until the person who suffers from such a condition realises it, because the feeling of pain in the abdomen is very slight.

Very few people aged over 50 in Western countries have normally-shaped intestines. If the pressure in the intestines augments because of blockages or gas, their shape changes. They distend in certain areas, lose their elasticity and become flabby; in other areas, they contract, become thinner and cramped. Often, their location also changes, and some parts of the intestines and the bowels shift to areas where they do not belong. The digestive organs lose their support and this allows them to be displaced. This again results in their malfunction; the abdomen becomes bloated and loses its shape.

BOWEL PROBLEMS

In the Western world, 40 to 50 per cent of the population suffers at least intermittently, sometimes chronically, from constipation. For women, the percentage is even higher – around 70 per cent. If the food is lacking in fibre, the nerve net which surrounds the large intestine is not sufficiently stimulated. In these cases, the nutrient solution often remains for days, sometimes even weeks, in the intestines, slowly becoming drier and drier. It is very possible that the person in question still goes once in a while to the toilet or even has diarrhoea, but even then, some of the excrement will keep sticking to the bowels. Fermenting excrement and other toxins create a very poisonous environment which can cause serious disease, such as colitis ulcerosa, diverticulosis or Crohn's disease. There is also the risk of re-intoxication in the upper intestinal regions. The root of many diseases is located in the intestines.

One of the most important tasks of the large intestine is to withdraw water from the nutrient solution so that the excrement in the colon will have the right consistency. Fibre normally keeps the excrement soft. If this is missing from the diet, constipation can easily develop. Coffee, black tea, cola and other soft drinks are dehydrating and worsen these problems in the long run. These drinks also irritate the kidneys, thereby withdrawing fluid from the body's water supply.

THE INFLUENCE OF THE INTESTINES ON POSTURE AND BACK PROBLEMS

(A Hypothesis of Dr Karl-Otto Heede)

Few people suspect that, for example, scoliosis (a curvature of the spine), spondylosis (back pain), lumbago and other back problems are often related to the condition of our digestive organs. A normal posture has become rare, and changes in the form of the thoracic cage (chest) are often the consequences of diseases of the abdomen, shifting of the organs and, above all, a constant pressure of gas in the abdominal cavity.

Without our being aware of it, this can release enormous forces, especially when this pressure always occurs in the same parts of the body. In these cases, first of all some of the lower vertebrae will be pressed slowly outwards, so that in the course of some years the waistline will spread and eventually disappear, a phenomenon which can be observed in most elderly people. In the case of a serious formation of gas in the abdominal cavity, any weak vertebrae, as well as the bones of the neck and the spine, can become dislocated and deformed. Even when people are still young, there can be a deviation of the spine because of this. Always, the organism will try to compensate for this by taking counter-measures, by drawing in part of the spine or by exerting a counter-pressure on the vertebrae. Consequently, lordosis, a hollow back, can develop, as well as spondylosis, scoliosis and other serious problems which can sometimes be very painful. Doctors try to cure these problems by using physiotherapy, bath treatments, gymnastics, chiropractic therapy, massage and different drugs – sometimes with, and sometimes without, success. When the abdominal cavity has not been thoroughly examined and the diseased intestines have not been treated, the physician can at best expect a temporary improvement, but nothing more.

Such treatments can take years, often many years, and all of them are insufficient if all the causes are not recognised and eliminated. Besides all these treatments, which are in themselves excellent, the most important thing would be to treat the original cause as well.

Dr Bircher-Benner, the renowned nutritionist, was very successful when treating patients who suffered from rheumatic diseases and problems of the spine by prescribing the right kind of diet. The wrong kind of nutrition – food which is lacking in many vital substances – weakens the muscles, the bones, the vertebrae and the spine.

THE WORST OFFENDERS

The following substances are mainly responsible for the shocking state of our health:

- Refined carbohydrates, such as sugar and flour
- Refined fats
- Additives
- Chemical residues from agriculture and stock breeding
- Chemical and synthetic drugs
- Addictive and unsuitable drinks

There is a clear connection between the intensive mechanical and chemical denaturalisation of our food and the typical diseases of our modern time. Every era has had its specific diseases, caused by the special conditions of the time. They depended on social, religious, economic, climatic and other environmental influences, as well as on the emotional lives of people during the period. The kinds of foods we eat are largely influenced by these elemental conditions. An inadequate and unbalanced diet, combined with other factors, has always been the basis upon which disease is able to develop.

Since prehistoric times, the type and composition of the food we eat has often changed, and people have always been able to adapt to these changes. When nothing else is available, man can live mainly on carbohydrates or animal protein for a long time, and he can survive on very little food. However, the ability of man to adapt is not unlimited. When natural food is processed ever more intensively and all the special ingredients which we need for our survival are removed, when natural products are turned into artificial products which have nothing in common with the original food, people cannot stay healthy. Therefore, on the following pages, I will describe in greater detail what effects the worst offenders have on our health.

Refined Carbohydrates

Sugar

Sometimes, health fanatics will tell you 'sugar is poison'. However, there is no need to regard sugar in quite such an extreme way. Sugar only becomes a problem when refined, industrialised sugar is used regularly, and, unfortunately, most people do this, often without realising it. This is because the sugar you eat comes not only from the sugar bowl but is also hidden in all kinds of food, even where you would never expect it to be.

Food manufacturers love to use sugar. In the first place, sugar is one of the best ways in which to preserve all kinds of food, as bacteria cannot live on such a processed substance. In the second place, they love to use sugar because it is addictive and everything prepared with some sugar sells extremely well. In former times, the sugar people consumed came from fruit, vegetables, tubers or roots. Honey was a rarity. In the fifteenth century, in tropical countries, sugar was extracted from sugar cane and exported in small quantities to Europe, but it was extremely expensive. Then, about 200 years ago, people learned to extract sugar from sugar beet. In the beginning, this procedure was very difficult and expensive, and for a long time sugar remained a luxury.

Today, everyone can afford to buy cheap, refined sugar, which is totally different from the natural product. Through extraction, heating, bleaching, etc., the manufacturers have produced an artificial, concentrated substance which contains hardly any of the vital nutrients we need, only calories. Sugar has been turned into a lifeless food which will damage our health if consumed regularly. This applies to any kind of sugar, perhaps with the exception of small quantities of natural honey or natural cane sugar, provided that both products have been treated in the old manner and have not been adulterated in any way. However, even of those, only minimal quantities are recommended, as such natural products themselves have a high concentration of sugars.

Sugar is a vitamin and mineral thief
When sugar is manufactured, all the fibre, vitamins and minerals contained in the original product are discarded. However, the human organism cannot metabolise sugar or any other refined food when these vital substances are missing. Therefore, minerals and other vital substances have to be confiscated from the body's own reserves, which can be found, for example, in our teeth and bones. Even small children who eat many sweets and pastries will suffer from dental decay.

For the same reason, many elderly people lose their teeth and, because of lack of exercise and bad eating habits, their bones become brittle and weak. Although nowadays in many homes for the elderly they serve a raw salad with or before the meal, coffee, a sweet dessert or a pastry is often served after it. This is a very bad custom, because refined sugar or flour in combination with raw salads will cause much fermentation in the intestines, stomachaches, flatulence and even more serious health problems.

The more sugar we eat, the greater becomes our lack of B vitamins, which are extremely important for our nerves. Nervous people and restless, sleepless children love sweets!

The blood sugar level and addiction to sugar

While in a healthy body the metabolism of sugar from fruit, raw vegetables and cereals which still contain all their original vital substances (vitamins, minerals, etc.) is never problematic, refined carbohydrates can cause a sudden steep rise in the blood sugar level, called hyperglycaemia.

The pancreas produces insulin, needed for the assimilation of sugar. However, in the case of refined sugar, the pancreas produces far too much insulin. In nature, sugar is always combined with fibre, vitamins, minerals and other substances, so our pancreas still produces the quantity of insulin needed for the digestion of sugar cane or big sugar beets, instead of producing only the insulin required for a small amount of sugar. After this sugar has been digested, there is still much insulin available, which should be used in some way. Now, the craving for something sweet starts, and, at the same time, the blood sugar level drops lower and lower. This condition is called hypoglycaemia and may cause extreme weakness, dizziness and fainting, or even circulatory failure.

The person affected thus will often go out of their way to obtain something sweet. As soon as they eat, for example, some chocolate, the craving abates, the level of sugar in the blood goes up and everything is fine until the now available sugar, in its turn, has been used. This can go on and on, and in this way a real addiction to sweets develops, which can be the cause of many serious diseases.

This again shows that any natural food which has been industrially manipulated has become an alien substance to the human body. It can disrupt normally well-balanced digestive processes, and cause functional disorders and many different diseases.

Wholemeal flour versus refined flour

All refined carbohydrates, such as sugar and refined flour (with the exception of freshly ground wholemeal flour), lack vitamins, minerals and other vital substances. These nutrients which are missing in such refined products are confiscated from the body's own supplies. If refined flour is combined with sugar, the body is deprived of still more vital nutrients.

For thousands of years, cereals were the staple food of most people. Cereal grains contain practically all the nutrients we need in order to be healthy. However, modern food technology manages to alter this and to manufacture completely useless products, which are the cause not only of obesity but also, amongst other problems, of constipation, from which, as I have said, as much as 50 per cent of the population of the Western world suffers.

Because our modern food contains ever-decreasing amounts of vital substances, sooner or later, the body's defences weaken. The acidity which occurs in the body when there is a lack of essential nutrients helps to produce all kinds of infections and the 'disease of civilisation'. B vitamins, which are lost during the refining of food, play an important role in the digestion of carbohydrates. When carbohydrates cannot be completely digested due to an absence of these vitamins, toxic substances accumulate in the body tissues and this can result in the development of malignant cells. In 2001, the WHO (World Health Organisation) linked the consumption of refined carbohydrates with a projected increase in several types of cancer in the next 10 to 20 years. This prediction has so far proved to be accurate.

These B vitamins are also important for the nervous system and the brain. People who eat many refined carbohydrates, especially children, are often extremely nervous. Furthermore, mental illness and Alzheimer's disease are on the increase in all industrial countries.

What About Fat?

Not so long ago, fat was a scarce commodity and was highly appreciated. Nowadays, everybody knows that we eat far too much fat. In North

America, the 'anti-fat movement' is an exaggerated reaction to the great problems with which the many obese people in that country have to cope. Research shows that 40 per cent of the American diet consists of fat, and now many Americans have a 'fat phobia' – they do not dare to eat the slightest amount of fat. This means good business for the food industry, and every supermarket and grocery store has started selling low-fat products, which they advertise in bold capital letters.

The average American citizen and many doctors are convinced that health problems such as obesity, heart and circulatory diseases, etc. are caused almost exclusively by the consumption of too much fat. This simply is not true! In believing this, one overlooks the important fact that sugar and other refined products, for example, are just as much to blame for the development of these diseases.

It is wrong and even dangerous to exclude every kind of fat from our nutrition – we need fat! Fats give us warmth and muscle power. Essential fatty acids are vital for the structure of our body cells and for their perfect function. Some vitamins cannot be utilised without fat. Fat has many important roles in our body.

Different kinds of fat

We do need fat, but not just any kind of fat. Some fats are good for us but some are bad for our health. The best fats are natural unsaturated and polyunsaturated fats, which we find in foods like avocados, nuts and oils which have not been treated industrially or changed in any way. However, as soon as these unsaturated fats are heated, they become saturated.

Natural unsaturated fats are, because of their biochemical structure, able to combine with natural proteins and thus play an important role in the transportation and utilisation of oxygen in our body. Such fats are easy to digest, whereas saturated fats can have the same kind of destructive effect on all organic functions as dangerous poisons.

They damage the red blood corpuscles as well as the composition of the blood, and in combination with too much protein, they can cause many chronic diseases such as diabetes, arteriosclerosis, cirrhosis of the liver and thrombosis.

Because of our polluted environment, some fats, particularly animal fats, contain highly poisonous fat-soluble chemicals such as insecticides, herbicides and detergents. These harmful animal fats, as well as synthetic fats, impair oxygen utilisation and respiratory processes, which are extremely important for a healthy metabolism. Of the animal fats, I can recommend only butter, as almost all kinds of margarine are lifeless industrial products and hardly ever contain healthy unsaturated fats. Butter contains many substances which are absolutely vital to our health. If, once in a while, you eat meat which contains some fat, it will not kill you. However, do not make a habit of this.

On the other hand, an avocado pear contains the right kind of fat, and you certainly will not gain any weight when you eat half an avocado with some lemon juice and no mayonnaise. Natural unsaturated oils, such as flax-seed oil and sunflower seed oil, lower the cholesterol content in the blood, prevent blood corpuscles from sticking together and lower the blood pressure. They help fight infections, prevent thrombosis and liver damage, and also have a soothing effect on the nervous system. Nervous, hyperactive children should regularly take some unsaturated oil – about two to three teaspoons daily.

You will find good unsaturated oils in health food shops. You should keep these in the refrigerator, as otherwise they soon become rancid. Vitamin C, magnesium, vitamin B and, above all, zinc are needed for the easy digestion of the healthy fat you need.

Food Additives

Until around 100 to 150 years ago, only natural ways of preserving food were known. Food was dried in the sun, in the air or at the fireplace, or was preserved by the use of sugar, salty or sour liquids, oil or starches. Later, preservation was achieved through heat and eventually by using very low temperatures or ice. When fruit and vegetables, for example, have not been changed by mechanical or chemical methods, freezing and drying are still the best and healthiest ways of preserving them.

However, as soon as fresh, natural food has been processed and adulterated by industrial manipulation in order to make it non-perishable, it becomes low-quality food which has lost all, or at least a great part, of its vital ingredients. Although some of these products still contain proteins, carbohydrates and fats, these have generally been changed to such an extent that they become worthless, harmful or even dangerous for our health when we eat them regularly. The preserving of food has become a very important commercial factor. About 80 per cent of all food in supermarkets today is either tinned or has been treated in one or more of many different ways in order to increase its shelf life or to improve its appearance.

When a natural product is processed, it loses its attractive appearance, its taste and its smell. Today, this is not a problem any longer. The chemical industry offers many substances which will enhance the taste and the smell of anything and can change even the most appalling-looking and -smelling food into a gourmet dream which says 'Buy me!' In 1950, about 700 such additives were already officially permitted. Today, there are over 4,000 additives available, which contain hardly any natural ingredients.

It is such a pity that our organism does not produce any digestive juices which can deal with additives! Many additives used to preserve food can paralyse or even kill bacteria or other very small creatures which happen to be in the food. People do not seem to know that bacteria and human cells are very similar: both of them have their own metabolisms and are highly sensitive to strong toxins. We may assume that such additives in our bodies would have a similar effect on human cells as they have on bacteria. However, nobody seems to worry about this and, as long as there is no proof that some of these additives are really dangerous for our health, the authorities will do nothing about them and their use will not be restricted. Every year, more people suffer from incurable diseases the causes of which are still unknown, and unless more research is undertaken, nobody will be able to prove that these have any relation to certain toxic substances which, for a great number of years, have been accumulating in the human body.

Many people, especially those responsible for the prosperity of industrial enterprise, point out that the extremely small quantities of additives being used are completely harmless, but there is now plenty of proof, for example in the case of homoeopathic remedies, that the human organism can react strongly to infinitely small quantities of toxic or non-toxic substances. Even Catherine de Medici killed her enemies using only the smallest amounts of poison!

The human body has not been equipped with anything which can detoxify the ever-growing quantity of foreign substances we take in day by day. Parts of these cannot be excreted and remain somewhere in the body, where they start to accumulate. These substances hinder metabolism as well as many other functions of the organism, and very little is known at present about what might happen when different toxins come into contact with each other, potentially causing dangerous inter-reactions. Although in medicine we have known about these problems for many decades, the industry completely ignores the fact that such reactions could be detrimental to our health.

As I have already made clear, one of the biggest factors in good health is correct digestion. We have to be careful that we give the body what is necessary, otherwise problems can occur. If food is not properly absorbed, then we encounter problems such as constipation or diarrhoea. What does one do in this day and age as a way of easing this inconvenience? Something that has become extremely fashionable and is often used is colonic irrigation. But is all this colonic irrigation necessary? Is it good for us? The reason I mention this is that, some time ago, one person told me that she did this every week! This made her bowels so lazy that they became ineffectual. It is essential that the friendly bacteria remain in the bowel when colonic irrigation is carried out. Not only the unwanted bacteria but also the good bacteria are often flushed out, so it is not advisable to undergo this procedure too often. I know we are able to encourage the growth of healthy bacteria with the use of acidophilus and biodophilus supplements, but this is still a big problem. I concur with all those people who are great believers in colonic irrigation and I know that cleansing the bowels periodically is beneficial, but certainly not every week and certainly not to the extent that one becomes addicted to this course of action.

Many years ago, when Alfred Vogel and I opened our first clinic for nature cure in Holland, an eminent professor approached us and asked if he could use our loft. When Vogel asked him why, he responded by saying that he wanted to set up some apparatus to show us what health was all about. He was busy for days putting it together and made a great job of it. He called this monstrosity he was building the 'higher bowel cleansing system'. He said that if we could refer a patient to him, he would demonstrate the process to us. A female patient agreed and was taken to him. The professor put her on this machine, proceeded to pump 20 litres of camomile water through her bowels and then showed us the end product – which consisted of almost half a bucket of waste material which had been flushed out. This made us realise not only how long the bowels are but also how much waste material accumulates there, which can often lead to more serious problems. Before leaving, the volunteer said she felt absolutely wonderful. So well, in fact, that the next day she returned and asked if she could have it again!

It is very true what my grandmother, who came from a long line of naturopaths, always said: a lot of diseases and illnesses make their home in the bowels. She would frequently prescribe castor oil as a means of cleansing them. It is therefore vital that we not only digest our food properly but also absorb it properly and then eliminate it properly. These are only a few valuable rules which are necessary to provide us with a great source of energy and also to encourage healthy living.

While I was sitting in the lounge of a well-known airline waiting to board a plane, I had a good look at a bored, overweight little gentleman sitting at the next table. Usually when one is bored, one looks for distractions by consuming the wrong type of food or drink. This man was a good example of this. He sat down, nervously took off his coat and then went straight to the bar. He came back with two bottles of wine and about four packets of small bagels, which vanished fairly quickly. He then returned to the bar and came back with six sandwiches, three packets of crackers and four small portions of cheese. These too were devoured. Even this did not alleviate his boredom, as he continued to puff and sigh as he waited to board his plane. So he went to the bar again, this time to reappear with two more bags of bagels, a cup of espresso coffee and two packets of food which, from a distance, I could not identify. While he was eating this, a quite unpleasant noise came from his table. He had problems with wind and flatulence, and was making loud burping noises. It was obvious to those around him that he wasn't feeling well. It was no surprise, given the time taken to consume all that food, not even chewing it properly or giving it a chance to mix with the saliva, that he felt unwell. Eating the combination of foods that he had in such a short space of time must have put tremendous strain on his system. When the flight was eventually called, he gradually stood up, made a few really unpleasant noises and then made his way to board the plane. As it was quite stormy during the flight, I wondered how he felt. He quite possibly arrived at his destination feeling extremely miserable and unwell.

We can certainly eat for comfort and do things that we shouldn't during periods of boredom, but is it really in order to do things that make us feel unwell and basically ashamed of our behaviour? We need to realise that by carrying out such actions we are attacking our digestive system and therefore it has a right to object. The nervous system is already working hard to cope with everyday stresses and tensions without having to contend with behaviour such as that I witnessed in the airport lounge.

It is common sense that the more relaxed we feel, the less nervous and tense we are. Life will become more enjoyable if we manage to handle things sensibly and with a little more care and attention.

CHAPTER TWO

Tips to Maintain a Healthy Weight

Every time I look at my book *Realistic Weight Control,* I appreciate how justified that book is today. When we consider the faddish slimming methods that have been used over the years, and also the methods that have been used to increase weight, they have all fallen by the wayside. In order to lose weight, we must adopt a whole new philosophy, a different lifestyle. Although some diets are probably moderately effective in their own way, we continue to live in a world with a tremendous number of overweight people. We all realise how unhealthy this is and for many people every single pound gained is a pound too many. I know the battle that people face and can fully understand how difficult it is.

Each day, I treat alcoholics as well as those addicted to nicotine and so on, and I have come to realise that addiction, especially to sugar, is an enormous problem. I recently saw a grossly overweight young woman who was drinking six bottles of cola per day. She was 23 years old and weighed 18 stone. Apart from feeling very uncomfortable and miserable, one could see that her brain was not functioning efficiently.

After examining her, I commented that her hair was lifeless, her nails were flaking and her liver was affected, and that something had to be done immediately to reverse this situation. What a job I had to get her mind to accept what she was doing wrong. We not only come across this problem with alcoholics and drug addicts, but also with those who are hooked on sugar, which is a particularly addictive foodstuff.

We now live in an era where the mind needs to be in control over what is wrong with our health. I see the great struggle that not only women but also men have to undertake in tackling this widespread problem of being overweight. Conversely, I also see the tremendous difficulties facing people who are underweight.

Balance is the key to these problems, but how do we overcome them? As I have often said, the spirit is very willing but the flesh is weak, and we often hear of those who have failed with tragic consequences. Being a diabetic, I understand the battle that people face, as I cannot afford to put on weight. Yet, when one puts one's mind to it, it can sometimes be easy. At a certain moment in my life, after my diagnosis with diabetes, my weight increased, but simply by dietary management I was able to lose two and a half stone in seven weeks.

The body is very complex, and it is necessary to understand how the metabolism works. One of the best methods of losing weight is to change one's diet immediately, and food combining is often of great help. In my case, being diabetic, I made a point of eliminating potatoes, bread, sugar, pasta and rice, and mainly consumed vegetables, fruits, fish and game, plus some rye bread for the slow release of sugar. In so doing, I established a diet whereby I lost all that weight – two and a half stone – in just seven weeks. So it can be done.

The other day, a lady stood on the scales in my clinic and told me in no uncertain terms that my scales were wrong. I told her that they were checked regularly, that they were right and she was wrong. To get that message across is sometimes very difficult but it is so important.

It is essential that we establish a good balanced diet. The one which Alfred Vogel and I created many years ago, which is detailed later in this chapter, is still very successful to this day.

First of all, you need to ask yourself if you really want to lose weight and what your motives are. We all know that being overweight causes a great deal of distress, all the more so because, in most cases, the sufferer is aware that the problem is of their own making. Many people go through life experimenting with diets. One week, it could be the 1,000-calorie diet, the next week could bring about the start of the vegetarian diet, followed by the even lower calorie diet or food combining. The life of the dieter can be extremely fraught. Of all the factors which can impede the progress of weight loss, the hardest thing to combat is temptation. This can creep up on you unawares: suddenly something sparks off a thought and you become obsessed with finding something particular to eat. This is very often for comfort, especially when you have other problems to cope with. Seemingly insignificant little habits can also have a great influence on your progress. Often, because of a lack of immediate success in dieting, people give up too quickly. Many find they are unable to stick to a diet unless they get some help and support. That can either come in human form (by means of treatment) or with the help of medication. However, one of the most important factors nowadays is exercise.

Don't make the mistake of promising that you will never eat anything sweet or fatty again, of saying you will never look at crisps or chocolate again, because you will. Realise that you cannot win every battle but you can achieve the ultimate victory. There will be plenty of excuses for throwing in the towel, but please do not succumb to them.

As I have observed, dieting is never easy. To assist you, I will therefore give you a few tips that I have mentioned in some of my previous books. Some people seem to set themselves up for failure before they have even begun. They go shopping and buy food as if it was going out of fashion. Everything that they could possibly need is bought in one go. In some ways, this can be useful for people who are dieting; on the other hand, if one has too much choice then deciding what to eat at a given moment becomes very difficult and, especially if one is hungry, this often leads to too much being eaten at once. The diet then fails before it has even started.

In order to prevent this kind of thing happening to you, I will provide you with a number of little tips which will help you through your daily life. A separate list is given for each of a number of situations which commonly give rise to problems, and these are followed by a list of general tips. As we have started by looking at shopping, the first of these lists deals with this subject.

SHOPPING

- Never shop on an empty stomach. If one is hungry, all sorts of temptations loom up in a supermarket.
- Before you set off on a shopping expedition, make a list of the things you need and don't look at anything else.
- Try to shop just once a week for the things on your list. If necessary, store them in the freezer.
- List your own food separately from the food that you are going to buy for the family.
- Do not buy your own favourite foods for the family. There are plenty of different foods on the market, so don't choose the ones that are going to tempt you the most.
- When you reach the checkout, try to concentrate on the person you are going to be once you are slim, and then you will not see all these tempting items most supermarkets keep just at the checkouts.

Having done your shopping and returned home, the next danger area you will enter is the kitchen.

IN THE KITCHEN

- Spend as little time as possible cooking. Don't go into the kitchen just to see what is there. Go in, do what you have to, then get out.

- While you are cooking, do not taste the food. A teaspoonful leads to a dessertspoonful, which leads to a tablespoonful, which really leads to a whole 'mini-meal' before you are even anywhere near the table. You know that your cooking is fine. You have probably been doing it for a long time, so there is no need to taste it!

- Whatever your particular diet, weigh all your food so that you know exactly what you are eating and how much.

- Do not allow yourself to be roped into baking or making toffee or fudge for good causes. There are plenty of other things that you could be doing for good causes, but do not make sweet things, because you know where some of them will go! There are enough people willing to do the cooking and baking who do not have a weight problem, or who are not concerned about their weight. Do something else, or even make a contribution so that someone else can do the cooking or baking, but do not do it yourself.

- Use cooking methods that do not entail a high number of calories. For example, food that is grilled is often much tastier than food that is fried in a lot of fat. Avoid frying and deep-frying as far as possible. Cook all your meat either by roasting, grilling or boiling. Be aware of how much fat you use in your cooking. Also be conscious of how much sugar you use. These are the calories that mount up rapidly without being particularly good for you. Food tastes much better in its natural state, so don't try to disguise it with a lot of fat or too much sugar.

Many of my dieters go out to work. This, again, is fraught with danger for someone trying to lose weight. So the next list concerns those who work away from home.

AT WORK

- Take a packed lunch with you. If you know exactly what is in your lunch, then you know that you are sticking to your diet. Hotels, restaurants and canteens cannot be held responsible for your gaining weight at lunchtime.

- It is a good idea to make your packed lunch well in advance. For example, perhaps on a Sunday evening you could make a week's supply of lunches in one fell swoop and then put them in the freezer. When you go out in the morning, take one packed lunch with you. It will not be thawed until lunchtime, so the temptation to eat it with your morning coffee will not arise.

- When coffee time arrives, do not be tempted by biscuits, scones, rolls or any other goodies that tend to be found in offices at that time of the day. Tell your colleagues what you are doing and then you will not dare to take something that you shouldn't in case they laugh at you.

- When you have eaten your lunch, find something to do that interests you, otherwise you may be tempted to go to the canteen for just that extra little something nice. Go window-shopping for clothes. Go to the library and read a book. Go for a walk. Do anything but expose yourself to more food.

- Do not keep sweets in a drawer. If you do, they will always be at the back of your mind and your will-power will fly out of the window. So see that there are no sweets, crisps or anything else around that might tempt you during working hours.

- Beware of office parties. In some large offices, every week there is at least one birthday party at lunchtime or at breaktime. If you have told your colleagues what you are doing, I'm quite sure they will not hold it against you if you refuse their piece of cake or their sticky bun or whatever treat they have brought because it is their birthday. Remember to refuse their offer politely but not regretfully. If you say 'no thank you' in a tone that really says 'yes please', then you will be coaxed, and inevitably you will be tempted and eventually accept the offering. If you are quite firm but still friendly, they will realise that your intentions are serious. They, in turn, will take you seriously and help you.

For some people, mealtimes at home present the greatest danger. Whether you are alone or in company, mealtimes can, for some people, be the cause of disaster.

MEALTIMES

- Always, even when you are alone, eat at the table, sitting in the same place. Eventually, you will come to regard this place as the only place in the house where you should eat.
- If you are having a hot meal, make your plate and your meal as hot as possible. This will help you slow down the rate at which you eat your food.
- Chew your food well. The more you chew it, the longer it will last and the more you will be satisfied. If you eat slowly, your stomach will tell you when you have had enough. If you eat too quickly, then although you have had enough, you will still feel hungry because your stomach has had no time to convey this full feeling to the brain.
- Put down your knife and fork between each mouthful. This is another way to make your meal last longer. If you eat it too quickly, then you will not feel you have had anything. This is where a warm plate and a piping hot meal come in handy. You do not need to rush to finish it before it is cold.

- Do not read at the table. While you are reading, your mind is only partially concentrating on what you are eating. Because of this, you eat mindlessly. You will then eat too quickly, with the result that you will eat too much.

- Eat your food from a smaller plate. Your meal will look more substantial if the plate is full. If your plate is too large, then your eye thinks you are not having enough to eat. So the fuller your plate, the more you are going to be satisfied with what you are eating.

- Do not finish off the family leftovers. This is a habit that many people are guilty of having. We all know about the starving millions, but eating up what your family leaves does not help them. All it does is prevent you from losing weight. If you have a dog or a cat, the problem is solved. If you have neither, I'm afraid the only solution is to throw it away. It is a waste, but perhaps in time you will learn that you are cooking too much food for your family. Cook them smaller meals if you frequently find that something is left over; but whatever happens, do not put the leftovers in your mouth.

For some dieters, having to socialise is the worst thing that can befall them. This need not be so. Remember, a social evening is not comprised solely of food. It is enjoying the company, the surroundings and the conversation. The food is provided simply as a means of making these things more pleasant. If you can view socialising in this light, then you will get the food into the right perspective. One does not go out solely to eat, rather one eats because one enjoys being with one's friends.

SOCIALISING

- When you are in a hotel, choose your meal sensibly.
- Remember to drink low-calorie, non-alcoholic drinks.
- Keep your glass full so that it cannot be filled up again.

- When you are eating, make sure, especially when at a friend's house, that you do not finish your meal first. That way you are less likely to be offered a second helping.
- If you are offered a second helping, do not accept it.
- Do not nibble aimlessly. When one is socialising, there are often all sorts of little nibbles available, but nobody minds if you do not partake of them.

For most people, the most difficult time of the day is the evening. They are in a relaxed mood and feel that they should have some sort of reward for having got through the hazards, trials and tribulations of the day. For many dieters, this reward means a treat that goes into the mouth.

EVENINGS

- Try to fill each evening with something that interests you. If you are bored when you come home from work and decide to do the ironing or the washing or clean the windows, then your mind will automatically turn to food. Find something that you think is stimulating and your mind will be occupied in a more constructive manner.
- It is good to get out in the evenings if possible. See if you can find an interesting evening class, go swimming or join a gymnastics or yoga class. I know that this is not always possible for those with children because there are times when nobody can look after them, but perhaps one or two evenings in the week can be filled in this way.
- If you are going to be at home in the evening, make sure that you have a dish of food that you are allowed to nibble on – food that is part of your diet – so that when you feel the urge to eat something, you are not spoiling a good day's work.
- Keep something back and have it for supper. If you have something

to look forward to, then the evening does not seem nearly so long. If you have your last meal at, say, six o'clock and know that no bite of food must pass your lips before breakfast the next day, then the evening can be very, very long, especially if food is in the back of your mind the whole time.

- One good way to resist temptation is to have a hot, luxurious bath and take a book with you.

- If you feel really tempted, it sometimes helps to clean your teeth. The feeling of needing something, especially something sweet, will usually pass. The same applies to having a cup of hot water and lemon juice. This also tends to take away the need for sweet things.

The tips given so far, if you heed them, should see you through the day. They all sound very good advice, and so they are, but sometimes they are not so easily followed. Temptation will, and does, creep in, so the next section will deal with such situations.

GENERAL TIPS

- When you have broken your diet, do not think that all is lost. If you have had a bad morning, then talk to yourself quite firmly but don't nag. That would just make you miserable. Don't try to starve yourself to make up for all the sins that you have committed, but just put them behind you and start afresh as soon as possible. When you break your diet on Monday, don't, like so many people, postpone your next dieting attempt for another week. Start right away, with the next meal, and you will find that by the end of the week you will still have managed some weight loss.

- The most discouraging part of any diet is when you come to a 'plateau'. You must persevere. Stop weighing yourself for a while and start measuring yourself. If you are truly sticking to your diet, then you will be encouraged. Remember, it is what you look like that counts

– it is the inches that you are losing that the world sees. They don't know every ounce that goes on or comes off your weight.

- Do not be envious of your thin friends who tend to eat far more than you do and never seem to gain an ounce. What these people are doing is storing up a fat future for themselves. At a later date, they will be most distressed to find that they can no longer eat the way they have been doing and stay slim. These people, when their sins catch up with them, will be far more miserable than the person who has had to diet throughout their whole life to keep anywhere near in trim.

- You will find that the outside world is not nearly as supportive of your diet as you think it should be. Dieting is a psychological process, not just for the dieter but also for those around him or her. For some reason, your slim friends may be afraid that you might catch up with them. Therefore, when they see a little weight coming off, they will tell you, 'You're all right, you don't need to go any further. You're slim enough.' Your fat friends will be discouraging too. They will see that you are doing what they ought to be doing and if they tell you, 'You're looking haggard. It doesn't suit you. Your disposition was much better when you were bigger,' there will be a fair measure of sour grapes. Don't listen to either set of friends. You will find that your most supportive friends are the ones who are trying to diet themselves. They will help and encourage you. They will be pleased with your weight losses and you, in turn, must be pleased with theirs. People who are not dieting tend to be very unsympathetic, either because they are thin and don't want you to be thin or because they are fat and don't want you to be thin.

- Sometimes you will find yourself in a situation you have not planned for. Knowing that these situations will inevitably arise, you must be ready for them at any given time. You may have planned your diet for the whole day and, suddenly, a very attractive invitation arrives for the evening. Always be aware that a situation like this may come up so that if you suddenly find yourself in a social position which you have not reckoned on, it won't throw you off your guard. You know the routine. Switch to it and stick to it.

- Every slimmer has a special time, or two or three times, in the day when dieting is particularly difficult. These times can take a person unawares, but you can work out when to expect them. The best way of dealing with this is by charting each day for a week. Write down everything that you eat and each time that you feel tempted. Note the emotion accompanying the temptation, or the situation in which you found yourself when the temptation struck. After a week, if you look at your chart, you will find that there is a pattern to it. There will have been certain times, certain emotions, certain situations, that triggered off a desire to binge. When you have determined which emotions and situations are likely to be dangerous, you can then sit down and make a campaign plan. How are you going to cope with them? If the problem is boredom, make sure that there is something to do at those dangerous times. If it is tension, try to do some relaxation exercises. If it is hunger – genuine hunger – make sure that you have something to eat, something that is already prepared and is part of your diet.

- When you are hungry, exercise. It is a fallacy that exercise makes you even hungrier. If you are active, you will find that the last thing on your mind is food. Activity has an exhilarating effect on the emotions. You feel alive, you feel fresh, you feel good and you don't want to spoil those feelings by being 'bogged down' with food. People only think that exercise makes them hungry. If you examine your feelings after having exercised, you will discover that, if you are honest, you have previously been conditioned to regard exercise as something that increases the appetite, whereas, in actual fact, the more one exercises, the less one wants to eat. So don't be afraid of moving. Don't be afraid of being energetic or exercising. It will give you a new lease of life and make you feel a lot better and much less hungry.

- Finally, I must talk here about vegetables. On most diets, these can be eaten freely – they certainly can on my diet. Some people seem to think that salad, like grapefruit, has a magical slimming quality. This, of course, is not true. Nevertheless, any vegetable prepared in any way other than frying will help your diet. I find that one good stand-by, and an excellent one for taking with you as a packed lunch, is slimmer's soup. There is no end to the varieties you can have. Basically, the recipe that I use is the same for each soup. You start with a stock cube and you can add anything that you like in the way of vegetables to it. Put in a tin of tomatoes, or tomato or vegetable juice, in order to give it some colour. Add to that anything you like: mushrooms, leeks, mixed vegetables. Don't be afraid of using herbs and spices, as they will give a richness to your vegetable soup. When the vegetables are tender, the soup is ready. At this stage, if you want to make a creamy soup, liquidise the mixture and add a little of your daily milk allowance. This will give you the feeling of eating a very rich soup, while in actual fact you can have as much of it as you like, because it is very low in calories.

- In winter, I find a very good way of making a satisfying vegetable soup is to make up a stock cube and add to your stock as many diced vegetables, fresh or frozen, as you want. When the soup is ready, liquidise half of it. This will make the stock much thicker and will fool you into thinking that you are eating something more substantial. Whichever way you like your soup, it is always tasty and is a quick, convenient, warming meal. You can have as much of it as you like, as many times a day as you like, so there is no excuse for saying, 'I broke my diet because I was hungry.'

These are methods that will always work, provided you work with them. They can make you feel less hungry and less tempted. It is up to you, however, to stick to your diet, and it is the degree to which you do this that determines whether you are going to lose weight. You get out of it what you put into it.

At the top of the diet sheet which follows, you will find a suggested day's menu. It should be stressed that this is just what it says – a suggestion. Underneath, there is a list of daily and weekly allowances, and this constitutes the diet. If you stick to your daily allowance and eat it within 24 hours, and if you eat your weekly allowance within seven days, then you are sticking to your diet. So just organise this to fit in with your own lifestyle. Don't try to change your lifestyle, but you must change your eating habits.

For example, if you are at work over lunchtime, take a weighed packed lunch with you. If you like something to eat before you go to bed at night, keep something back. If you are working during the night, eat your allowances over a 24-hour period. If you are a nibbler, then you are allowed to nibble, as long as what you nibble is on the diet sheet and weighed as part of your allowance.

Don't take any fewer than three meals per day. It is not a good idea to take your allowance in one fell swoop, as you will overload your stomach and your metabolism will not work. One large meal will lie there like a great log on an empty fire, and no amount of matches will get that log burning. What your body needs is light meals, several times per day. Each time you eat, you speed up your metabolism slightly. So six small meals a day will give you this little extra boost six times instead of the normal three.

Before you start, read the diet below carefully and get yourself organised. Shop for the things that you will want for the next few days. See to it that everything you need is in the house, so that you will not be tempted to reach for the biscuit tin. See to it when you are out working that there is something ready to have when you come in. That does not mean to say that your hot meal has to be ready when you come home, but see to it that you have a 'nibble dish' in the fridge consisting of various sorts of vegetables, again so that you will not automatically reach for the wrong foods.

WEIGHT REDUCTION DIET
Suggested Day's Menu

Breakfast: fruit

egg (poached, boiled, scrambled, omelette)

wholewheat bread or toast, plus butter (or exchange)

Mid-morning: tea or coffee

Lunch: lean meat, fish, egg, cheese

vegetables or salad

wholewheat bread or toast plus butter (or exchange)

fruit

tea or coffee

Mid-afternoon: tea or coffee

Evening Meal: clear vegetable soup or tomato juice

lean meat, fish, egg, cheese

vegetables or salad

wholewheat bread or toast, plus butter (or exchange)

fruit

tea or coffee

Bedtime: decaffeinated tea or coffee, or herbal tea

Allowances

Daily: milk: fresh – ½ pint/300 ml; or powdered
                  – 1 pint/600 ml
               wholewheat bread – 3 oz/90 g
               meat – 4 oz/120 g; or fish – 6 oz/180 g
               fruit – 3 portions
               cheese – 1 oz/30 g

Weekly: butter or margarine – 4 oz/120 g
               eggs – 7

Exchanges for 1 oz/30 g Bread

potato – 1 medium
crispbread, crackers, water biscuits – 2
breakfast cereal – 1 oz/30 g, any sort except sugar-coated varieties
cooked rice – 2 dessertspoonfuls
plain biscuits or oatcakes – 2

Variety is the spice of life: choose your allowances from these foods

Meats
4 oz/120 g daily, cooked any way except fried

Beef, chicken, corned beef, duck, kidney, lamb, liver, mutton, rabbit, sweetbreads, tongue, tripe, turkey, veal

Fish
6 oz/180 g daily, cooked any way except fried

Cod, crab, haddock, hake, halibut, herring, kipper, ling, lobster, mackerel, mussels, oysters, pilchards, prawns, salmon, sardines, shrimp, trout, tuna

Eggs

7 per week

Poached, boiled, scrambled, omelette

Although seven a week are allowed, if you are trying to lower your cholesterol it would be advisable to eat fewer.

Cheese

1 oz/30 g daily

Caerphilly, Camembert, Cheddar, Cheshire, Danish blue, Edam, Gruyère, Leicester, Parmesan, Roquefort, smoked Austrian, Stilton, Wensleydale

4 oz/120 g daily

Cottage cheese

Vegetables

Unlimited

Artichokes, asparagus, aubergines, beans (French and runner), bean sprouts, beetroot, Brussels sprouts, broccoli, cabbage (red, Savoy, spring, winter), carrots, cauliflower, celery, chicory, courgettes, cress, cucumber, lettuce, marrow, mushrooms, onions, parsley, parsnips, peppers (red, yellow and green), pickles (dill, gherkins, red cabbage), pimentos, radishes, spinach, spring onions, swede, tomatoes

In moderation

Avocado (no more than half a day), baked beans (no more than 3 ½ oz/ 105 g a day), beans (butter, broad, haricot), peas, sweetcorn

Fruit

3 portions daily – portion sizes given below

    apple, 1 average

    apricots, 2 fresh

    banana, 1 small

    blackberries, 4 oz/120 g

    cherries, 4 oz/120 g

    cooking apple, 1 large, baked or stewed

    damsons, 10

    dates, 1 oz/30 g

    gooseberries, 10

    grapefruit, 1 large

    grapes, 3 oz/90 g

    juice, 3 ½ fl. oz/100 ml, unsweetened

    melon, 1 slice

    orange, 1 average

    peach, 1 average

    pear, 1 average

    pineapple, 1 slice fresh

    plums, 2

    pomegranate, 1

    raisins, 1 oz/30 g

    raspberries, 4 oz/120 g

    rhubarb, 4 oz/120 g

    strawberries, 4 oz/120 g

    sultanas, 1 oz/30 g

    tangerines, 2

Drinks

Unlimited

Bovril, coffee, herbal tea, low-calorie tonic, Marmite, Oxo, slimline drinks, soda water, tea, tomato juice, water

Tea and coffee should not be taken with sugar, and if milk is added, it should be subtracted from the daily allowance.

Seasonings

Unlimited

Herbs, lemon juice, mustard, pepper, salt, spices, vinegar, Worcestershire sauce

These foods are best avoided

Sugar and its products

Chocolate, commercial milk drinks, glucose, ice cream, jam, lemonade, lemon curd, marmalade, puddings, squashes, sweetened yoghurt, sweets, syrup, tinned fruit, treacle

Fatty foods

Black pudding, chips, cream, crisps, dripping, fishcakes, fish fingers, fried foods, lard, oil, roast potatoes, salad cream, sausages

White flour and its products

Bridies, buns, cakes, crumpets, doughnuts, dumplings, packet soups, pasta, pastries, pies, sausage rolls, scones, sweet biscuits, thickened gravies, sauces, pickles, chutneys and soups

Miscellaneous items

Alcohol, artificial sweeteners, diabetic foods and squashes, evaporated or condensed milk, honey, nuts, processed meat, slimming biscuits

Many people come to me maintaining that they cannot lose weight, the reason being 'I work' or 'I work at nights', or 'the canteen at work doesn't cater for slimmers'. These are feeble excuses. If you work, you are one of the privileged ones. If you work at night, then it doesn't matter. The diet allows you to take your daily allowance over a 24-hour period. You must have a meal at night, otherwise while you are working your blood sugar will become too low, and then you will not be able to work responsibly. The food at work cannot be held responsible for your failure to lose weight. You are responsible for this, so don't blame the canteen – don't go to it. When you are out working, take a weighed meal with you so that you know exactly what you are consuming.

Some people see obstacles everywhere, and they generally find that they do not lose weight. They are so busy looking at the difficulties that they forget to do their part – the simple part of organising themselves to give themselves a good chance of losing weight.

The diet I have detailed in this chapter is a good standard diet, but there are many problems concerning weight that have to be looked at individually.

LOW BLOOD SUGAR

The other day, I saw a lady who had tried everything to lose weight. She had been to every slimming clinic there was, but nobody could pinpoint why she could not shed any weight. It was not until she consulted me that it became clear that she had a low-blood-sugar problem. It is vital that the blood sugar level is controlled, as low blood sugar can often lead to many physical and mental problems. However, this lady's problem was easily solved with the introduction of chromium, which also combated her cravings for chocolate – her favourite foodstuff. As soon as her blood sugar level was controlled with chromium, she managed to lose weight. Administering chromium to young children who have become addicted to chocolate can have a beneficial effect too.

Many physical and mental problems are caused by low blood sugar (hypoglycaemia). This is a disturbance in the metabolism of sugar. Low blood sugar is a widespread condition, even in the smallest of children, and often goes unrecognised. A child can be categorised as listless, with no interest in school, or easily distracted and unable to maintain concentration on a subject, when in fact their brain is incapable of functioning properly due to insufficient fuel.

Some well-meaning parents are still under the impression that sugar of any kind is good for the brain. 'The brain needs sugar, and my child eats a good deal of sugar,' a loving parent might say. But that is exactly the problem. What the brain needs continually, besides oxygen, is glucose, not sucrose. After someone consumes food or beverages containing industrial sugar (i.e. sucrose), their blood sugar level will soar within minutes. Then the pancreas will supply insulin, needed for the digestion of this sugar. Soon the job will be done – the sugar will be digested, and usually after one or two hours or even sooner, the blood sugar level falls far below normal. This triggers an immediate craving for more sweets or soft drinks, and the process will be repeated.

Frequent consumption of food or beverages containing refined sugar can easily induce hypoglycaemia as an almost constant condition. As a consequence of chronic low blood sugar, the normal functions of the pancreas are disturbed. Because of this, hypoglycaemia is often a preliminary stage of hyperglycaemia (high blood sugar) and diabetes, which has lately been increasing at a frightening speed all over the world. If people with these conditions do not change their eating and drinking habits, they will suffer. Some starchy foods, like wholegrain cereals, will maintain a steady level of blood sugar, whereas starches like white bread, white rice and white noodles can be responsible for excessive variations in the blood sugar level, although not ones as extreme as those caused by refined sugar.

It was amazing how much weight the lady I mentioned above lost on *Helix Slim,* a remedy first produced by Alfred Vogel, with chromium and a well-balanced protein-based diet. She saw remarkable results, losing 4½ stone. At her initial consultation with me, she had weighed 21 stone.

GUIDELINES FOR SLIMMING WITHOUT DANGER

Obese people must never let themselves be persuaded to take a commercial slimming product. Never take an ordinary preparation that contains iodine, since iodine is a dangerous element and should be used only in homoeopathic potencies and with the greatest caution. So, if you do not know the contents of a slimming product, be sure to find out and reject it if it contains iodine. Seaweed is an exception, because it contains a natural iodine which is very quickly absorbed. One should be very sceptical of any highly publicised weight-reducing remedies. Remember, the safest way to lose weight is by means of a suitable diet and a well-planned programme of physical therapy.

All chemical slimming preparations should be completely avoided. They are dangerous, not only to the health but to life itself. Some people who have taken these preparations have met a tragic end. If you feel you must lose weight, take nothing but natural remedies. In this way, the natural way, the problem of obesity will be solved much more effectively.

BODY WEIGHT AND THE ENDOCRINE GLANDS

When deciding how to approach a problem of obesity, it is first necessary to identify its cause. It is no doubt true that excess weight is often caused by an improper diet or by eating too much. In most cases, whether the patient was underweight or overweight, it was thought in the past that the cause was the intake of food. However, there are some people who eat a lot and remain extraordinarily thin and others who eat very little and still put on weight. These people cannot control their weight simply by changing the amount of food they consume.

Research has shown that dysfunction of the endocrine glands, the glands responsible for internal secretions, is largely responsible for both excessive corpulence and thinness. These glands are, primarily, the pituitary, the ovaries, the testicles and the thyroid. Their overactivity, or imbalance, usually leads to thinness, while their underactivity, or insufficiency, leads to corpulence.

Those who put on weight although they eat very little suffer from impaired functioning of the endocrine glands. In my medical practice, I have observed cases where the gonads, as well as the pituitary glands or the thyroid, were responsible for obesity. If such functional disorders have been ongoing since youth, the gonads are generally underdeveloped or retarded as far as proper activity and hormone production is concerned. In such cases, fat is often deposited on the hips and waist only and never on the arms and legs, so that these limbs are not excessively big. In women, the breasts show considerable fat deposits instead of being the shapely glands they normally are. Sagging breasts, due to a malfunction of the ovaries, are often an additional worry of overweight women. This type of obesity cannot be dealt with successfully by either dieting or any other kind of slimming course. Weight loss may be possible only if the causes are treated.

It has been observed that removal of the ovaries, or diseases causing ovarian insufficiency, result in a woman putting on weight. Obesity brought on by the menopause confirms the truth of this statement. Typical examples are the inhabitants of southern climates. How slim and supple the Italian or the Latin and South American girls are in the early prime of life. But as soon as the glandular secretions diminish, which is usually at a much earlier age in hot countries, they become plump. If the older generation is stout, solid and comfortable, the reason for this can be traced to the insufficient functioning of the endocrine glands and, more than anything else, sluggishness of the ovaries. In such cases, sitz-baths (therapeutic hip baths) and other therapies which stimulate the ovaries would be of immense help towards reducing corpulence. The remedy *Ovarium,* in combination with a good diet, has also given good results.

Another simple method of stimulating the ovaries is to take various foods that contain vitamin E. The most important of these is wheatgerm. There are some people who will not eat wheatgerm for fear of getting fat, because it is also been recommended to thin people who wish to gain weight. Women need not worry about this, since wheatgerm and its vitamin E content only regulate the function of the ovaries. In fact, wheatgerm stimulates their function in the case of fat people and reduces their overactivity in the case of thin people. In this way, it actually helps the obese to lose weight and the thin to put it on. In addition, wheatgerm contains other valuable nutrients, such as vegetable protein, phosphates and natural sugar, all of which have a good effect on the body without the danger of causing an abnormal weight increase. So, if you suffer from obesity, do not hesitate to eat wheatgerm, for it will not increase your weight, but regulate or control it.

For the obese, wheatgerm oil should be supplemented with *Kelp,* a seaweed preparation, so that the thyroid and other endocrine glands will also be stimulated. The body weight will be regulated and the general condition of health improved without the patient having to follow a strict diet. Excessively thin people too can normalise their weight with the help of wheatgerm oil. With underweight people, where there is a problem with the endocrine glands, it is a good idea to take a few remedies, such as *Ovarium* or *Centaurium* twice a day, in order to balance the system. My book *Menstrual and Premenstrual Tension* gives in-depth advice on this.

Pituitary obesity, however, is not so easy to deal with because the pituitary is less amenable to corrective treatment than the ovaries. There are, of course, glandular preparations on the market which do act on the pituitary, but their administration is still a delicate matter. Nor do these preparations always produce positive results with the pituitary, though they often do with the ovaries. A more effective way to reduce pituitary obesity is to take the seaweed ocean kelp. Two *Kelp* tablets taken twice a day are usually enough to reduce excess weight slowly but surely. Additionally, take *Helix Slim*, a fresh plant extract made from *Helianthus tub*, over a long period of time.

THE ENDOCRINE GLANDS AND THE MIND

In order to overcome the widespread problem of obesity, we first of all have to be aware of how the mind really works. Frustrations, fear and other negative mental states finally result in crystallised matter at the negative pole of the body (the pelvic basin). This is because the mind affects the glandular areas, which carry out energy distribution in the body. These, like a spinning wheel, whirl from the right and increase in their circumference, thus energising five zones on each side of the body, the right and left. The downward thrust constitutes a line which transverses the entire body, back and front, and so also does the upward thrust. Hence you have five lines on each side of the body. Each zone line passes through different portions of the anatomy.

In therapy, the positive, negative and neuter poles are most important. The vital thing is that the energy from the positive pole is able to reach the negative pole. As in good health, this is the rhythm of life. Mental upsets, dietetic errors and all the other factors which modern civilisation has thrust upon us prevent this in varying degrees. The positive pole (the head) is short-circuited, like the fuse box that controls a lighting system. Energy piles up at the negative pole as a result. People can suffer from varying degrees of ill health – acute and chronic states. The life-giving energy can also be blocked in varying degrees – where it gets blocked entirely, death is the result.

The real skill of the therapist comes in finding just where these blocks are and connecting the system up again so that the body current can flow from the head to the feet in a normal way. This is the key to many medical riddles. Acupuncture is a terrific help here. I have had tremendous success over the years in bringing patients' systems back into balance using acupuncture. In patients who are overweight, acupuncture can successfully be used to balance the positive and negative to a level where the mind can then control any bad eating or drinking habits. Furthermore, exercises such as yoga, Alexander technique or Pilates are of the greatest help.

Where there is an imbalance in the endocrine system, one can also do a tremendous amount to help by the use of cranial manipulation. It is quite interesting to see how, by the use of cranial work, one can influence the pituitary gland, which controls the metabolism and can quite easily cause problems with being either overweight or underweight.

Body endocrine balance on the cranium can work very well. I have included a chart here and an explanation of how it works.

If you visit a trained practitioner who is able to apply the simple technique of energy balance to the endocrine zones on the human skull, miracles can be made to take place. No harm can ensue from an endocrine energy balance treatment. It is not like taking drugs or hormone extracts – this method will only excite the glands to function, not to over-function. If some of the glands do over-function, this same simple technique will bring the glands back to normal.

The endocrine zones of the skull are tied up with those of the feet. The therapist uses the thumb of the right hand on the left foot and the thumb of the left hand on the zones of the cranium.

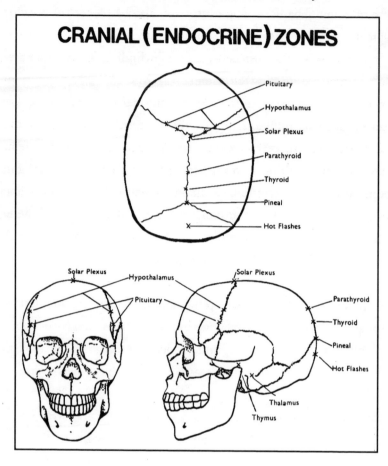

The endocrine reflex zones of the cranium

After doing this for a few minutes, they will change over and apply the opposite hands, in other words the thumb of the left hand to the zones of the right foot and the thumb of the right hand to the cranium zones.

In this way, pure and simple energy balance can be initiated by the application of the thumbs. I wrote more about this particular type of work in my books *The Five Senses* and *Body Energy*.

The question remains, 'Is there any easy way to balance body weight?' Where people are overweight, it is a matter of focusing the mind, which is stronger than the body, and following a good balanced diet, such as that detailed in this chapter. There are also some wonderful remedies available, such as *Helix Slim, Api Slender* and *Fat Metabolism Factor,* which all offer extra help, as does acupressure or acupuncture. But above all, remember that whatever the reason for being overweight, the problem should be investigated, otherwise health can suffer. A good, healthy programme, like the many methods I have described in this chapter, will be of great assistance. On the other hand, being underweight is very often a question of equilibrium. Success mostly lies in balancing the endocrine system and, as I have mentioned, try using remedies such as *Centaurium,* sometimes with the addition of zinc or possibly some chromium. In addition to this, sensible exercise, together with a dose of common sense, will help you on your way. As I often say, there is nothing common about common sense.

CHAPTER THREE

How to Beat Addictions

Many people are addicted in one way or another. Some don't even know that they are. There are various forms of this disease: there is addiction to bread, chocolate, ice cream, coffee, alcohol, drugs, sweets or cola drinks. Some addictions are more dangerous than others, but none is harmless. Some addictions which are related to nutrition can be caused by a malfunction of the pancreas, but all addictions have the same origin. Addicted people yearn for something they miss or lack, not only emotionally but also physically. For instance, why does a person become an alcoholic? Some people who have a personal problem start drinking to calm down. Emotional problems give the first push towards addiction, and many doctors still believe that psychological problems and too little will-power are the only causes.

That addictive behaviour can also have physical causes is not well known. Although some people may drink once, twice or three times too much because they have a personal problem, only a small percentage of these people become really addicted to alcohol. Why does one person become an alcoholic and another person not? It is certainly not a question of character. The problem lies elsewhere.

The need for certain nutrients is different with every person. There are people who need a lot more of some vitamins, minerals or vital substances than others. Many people, even if they eat healthy food, often cannot assimilate or store these vital nutrients. In order to assimilate and process alcohol, coffee, sweets or – even in the case of non-smokers – cigarette smoke, the organism uses up great amounts of vital nutrients.

When a person who leads a healthy life (if that is still possible in this day and age) drinks a little too much from time to time, it won't harm them. However, if somebody else who suffers from a chronic lack of vital nutrients does the same, they will become an alcoholic sooner or later, depending on the state of their health. With every glass of wine or every cigarette, a greater desire develops which cannot be met in the long run. The person concerned feels that they lack something and becomes nervous and restless. Then they will again reach for the glass, a cigarette or drugs, and the vicious circle continues. In this way, the person in question gets deeper and deeper into the addiction.

Many of these people will be convinced by their physician or by their friends that their addiction stems only from their weak character. Because of this, they often go into deep depression and, over and over again, they succumb to their addiction. It is hardly possible for them to get out of this vicious circle by themselves. One cannot do it alone.

The origins of addiction are difficult to pinpoint. It all starts in the cradle or even before children are born. Addictive behaviour inherited from parents, or learned from the consumption of sweets, soft drinks and junk food – and the resulting restlessness, hyperactivity or autistic behaviour – lies at the bottom of the increasing tendency towards addiction.

From kindergarten on, children can get into the quicksand of ever-escalating temptations, and in order to get them out of the spiral of addiction, we must change our own attitudes in a very drastic manner. We all have a tendency to put the blame for the present sad situation on other people. We blame the cigarette and alcohol industries, publicity, television and drug cartels. Of course, all of those do a lot of harm; nobody who loves their children will deny this. But we should keep in mind that all business is always a question of supply and demand; whenever products are sold successfully, it means there is a great demand for them.

ALCOHOL

A few weeks ago, as I was nearing the end of my appointments for the evening, a charming, intelligent psychiatrist sat before me. This young lady was so dedicated to her profession that, in an attempt to help her patients, she would carry the weight of their problems on her own shoulders. This put her under tremendous stress and, as a means of trying to alleviate the pressures of the day, she gradually turned more and more to having that extra glass of whisky, vodka or brandy. By taking that course of action, she said, she felt more relaxed, which, in turn, made her feel better. However, she admitted that what had started as a small problem had escalated into an addiction. As we chatted, she realised that I totally understood the immense pressures she was under on a daily basis. I concurred that life is extremely difficult nowadays; I too see patients who are very demanding and who virtually expect an overnight miracle when they are faced with health problems. In times like this, when one is depressed, being offered comfort and support can work wonders.

How many people have abused alcohol as a way of relieving stress and unwittingly become addicted? Alcohol can be a real enemy. We often make light of those people who prefer to turn to that extra drink as a way of relaxing, instead of resorting to some tranquillising drug, not realising that this can ultimately be their ruination. I have often seen those who thought they had won the battle and, because of their achievement, felt it would do no harm to celebrate with just one little drink.

When I first arrived in Scotland, over 40 years ago, and caught a bus from Waverley Station in Edinburgh to my destination, I realised that the people of Scotland took drink very much for granted. It was just after Christmas, and we drove past a man on the street hanging around a lamp-post, completely drunk. On seeing this, the bus conductor said to the driver, 'Look at him,' to which the driver answered, 'Well, well, what a pity. Never mind, next week it'll be my turn.' What a lot of people fail to understand is that what can be just a pleasant drink for many can lead to destruction in others.

If my young psychiatrist patient had not managed to stop, she would have gone down that road because, even in those as intelligent as she is, the mind becomes uncontrollable and one doesn't know what to do next or where to turn for help. We have to use will-power and even force to overcome the problem of addiction. One should never be afraid to accept help whenever it is available, whether it be through Alcoholics Anonymous (AA) or a doctor or psychiatrist.

Many people have ended up in the gutter or even in prison because they rejected help. I reflect on some of my failures and where they are today. One man I dearly loved, who was commended for his help in the community and to others, lost his battle with alcohol. He could not conquer the problem he had with drinking. I agree with those doctors who say that alcohol causes brain damage. By the time the problem has reached a serious stage, the individual concerned is often incapable of thinking clearly and will do things which are totally out of character. It is so sad that those in desperate need of help often decline it. This particular gentleman was full of good intentions but could no longer cope. He once told me that when any problem surfaced, he tried to blank it out. When bills came in, he would hide them and, like the ostrich, he would put his head in the sand, trying to forget about them by having another drink.

This brings to mind one of my dearest friends. As we had been close friends for such a long time, I felt it would be more appropriate for him to seek independent help and I repeatedly advised him to do so. Although I managed to find someone who was well qualified to help, that professional could not get through to my friend. He had a large, successful business but ended up in the gutter. I had another acquaintance who I repeatedly warned. He became uncontrollable and ended up in prison. As I have said, alcohol can be a real enemy, as I have seen too often in my lifetime.

The other night, I took a call from a wonderful lady. She and her husband are devoted to each other and their children. She phoned me after finding a text message on her husband's mobile to a former friend of his – or, to be precise, an ex-lover. She was distraught and on the point of leaving him. Because it had been a text message, I suggested that we delve deeper into it. So, that evening, I went to see them both. It became evident that her husband had been totally drunk when he sent this message to his former lover which nearly destroyed their happy marriage. Fortunately, they were able to sort things out because she was aware that he had acted in a way which was completely out of character. These are just a few examples of problems that can occur through misuse of alcohol.

Stress is a great problem. We often lift up a glass in stressful situations and toast to 'Good health and happiness'. But when happiness is driven further and further away through lack of determination to stop drinking, then what starts off as just one problem soon spirals out of control, leading to even bigger ones.

At the time of writing this book, the headlines in the newspapers are dominated by similar problems facing a great politician, the former leader of the Liberal Democrat Party, Charles Kennedy. He had a bright future before him, but was forced to resign dramatically due to his drink problem and was left contemplating the ruin of his 23-year career. He not only used his resignation speech to plead for party unity but also to reproach some of his own MPs for failing to stand by him through his crisis. This is an example of what can happen when stress becomes too great to bear and when, possibly, one is given too little help to overcome the problem.

Alcohol has a long tradition in our culture. In the past, people liked to drink during festivities and sometimes they drank excessively. However, following these feast days, there were long periods when there were no financial means to afford this 'party drinking'. All this has changed. Now, certain foods and specific drinks are kept for special occasions, while beer, wine and other alcoholic drinks have become a daily pleasure. They are served all the time and everywhere. In the last 40 years, statistics show, the consumption of strong alcoholic beverages has increased threefold. The quantity of beer drunk has increased by four and people now drink five times as much wine as before. The consequences are known.

The future looks bleak as far as alcohol abuse is concerned. Even today, we see many young boys and girls with problems and one reads in the national papers of how alcohol consumption is the cause of countless crimes. Many children as young as 11 and 12 start experimenting with alcohol, and surveys show that their most popular drinks are beer, lager and cider, and sometimes spirits. Fizzy alcopops have become very popular and usually the alcohol content of these drinks is quite high. In 1986, just 20 children were treated at Alder Hey Hospital in Liverpool for alcohol intoxication; by 1996, this figure had increased tenfold to 200. The hospital in Liverpool reported that children as young as eight were being admitted with acute alcohol intoxication. In one survey, more than half of 14-year-old schoolchildren in Scotland reported having been drunk. This increase in cases was not restricted to Liverpool. Figures from accident and emergency units across the country suggest that around 50,000 teenagers are now being admitted with acute alcohol intoxication each year.

Children drink mainly to alter their mood or cope with stress, because they want to feel happy and forget their problems – this is much easier when the brain is numbed. By drinking alcohol, they also bond with friends, and the exploring of sexual relations becomes easier. Alcohol-related problems include reduced performance at school, quarrels and arguments, sexual problems, fights, vandalism, driving accidents and many different health concerns. When drinking is combined with smoking, health risks are still greater. Evidence shows that alcohol misuse while young is associated with heavy and problematic drinking in later life. There is also an association between alcohol abuse – especially heavy drinking during teenage years – and the use of illegal drugs.

By and large, children follow their parents' example. Heavy-drinking parents tend to produce children who misuse alcohol. Excessive consumption of drink in adolescents may be related to low levels of parental support and control. About five years ago, an American report found that underage drinkers are four times more likely to develop alcohol dependence than those who begin drinking at the age of twenty-one.

Even those who are not actually dependent on alcohol can be inviting serious problems. Many people today appear to be under the impression that they can drink as much as they like without any adverse effects. Unfortunately, binge drinking can cause brain damage. The binge drinker takes the risk that the brain might be harmed and, as new research suggests, these people are in as much need of treatment as alcoholics are for their addiction. According to newspaper reports, heavy social drinkers show the same pattern of damage as alcoholics, to the extent that their day-to-day lives are impaired. Scans carried out on people who drink more than 100 units of alcohol per month (equivalent to 50 pints of lager or 100 glasses of wine) revealed some degree of brain damage. The Government has now realised that much has to be done to curb binge drinking.

This book is all about health and vitality. Health suffers as a result of the intake of alcohol, and each drop will affect not only the brain cells but also the liver. Many people, particularly alcoholics, seem to feel that their vitality and energy levels increase when they drink. In fact, the opposite happens. I have seen so many problems of toxicity of the liver that I have had to use strong antitoxins, like Vogel's *Detox Box,* and a strong antioxidant such as *Daily Choice Antioxidant* or even a blood detoxification remedy from Michael's, *Blood Detoxification Factors.* Help is at hand if you want to take it.

A young man came to see me who had made great progress for a while but who, somewhere along the road, had lost all motivation to live. He had a brilliant brain, but as a consequence of the stresses and strains of life, he went downhill and could not control the enormous problems he had with alcohol. I talked to him in the middle of the night and told him that we would fight his alcohol addiction together. Acupuncture helped him tremendously and, with the addition of homoeopathic remedies, plus huge doses of vitamin C and ginseng to boost his system, I am happy to say that today he has attained a high position as a professor in mathematics. So, yes, there can be help for this massive problem which nowadays we call alcoholism.

I often hear people say that their lives would be boring if they drank no alcohol. Although some people find the truth difficult to take, alcohol should only be drunk in small quantities. In small amounts it is not harmful to healthy adults. There are many controversial ideas about how much one should drink. A unit of alcohol is defined as 10 ml of pure alcohol. It is recommended that men drink no more than three or four units per day, the approximate equivalent of two glasses of wine. A woman's liver does not tolerate alcohol as well as a man's and the limit for women is slightly lower. It is best not to drink alcohol every day. Your liver needs a rest in order to recover. It should be mentioned that the quantity of alcohol considered 'safe' has been lowered each year since the guidelines were brought in. It is quite possible that, in the future, alcohol will be seen in a more critical light.

Many people are of the opinion that it would be boring not to drink alcohol or to reduce it to such a low level, but adhering to these rules will offer protection against becoming an alcoholic. From the moment one becomes an alcoholic, not another single drop can be taken without serious consequences.

COFFEE AND OTHER ADDICTIVE DRINKS

I am often asked if there is anything safe to drink. Of course, it is necessary to drink, but there are addictive drinks as well as drinks that are good for us. Many people nowadays prefer to drink coffee, black tea, hot chocolate, soft drinks, cola drinks and perhaps some milk, which is often quite indigestible, instead of water. Since the First World War, the consumption of coffee and sweet drinks has increased tenfold.

Coffee and other drinks containing caffeine stimulate the taste buds in the mouth. They also stimulate the digestive juices in the stomach, increase the heartbeat and the functions of the brain, help temporarily against migraine headache and stimulate urine production and bowel movement. These reactions may last only a few minutes or sometimes several hours. Then the counter-reaction starts. The coffee drinker becomes more and more nervous and sometimes shaky, melancholic or depressive. Habitual coffee drinking can be the cause of serious or chronic migraines.

Sugar addiction and coffee addiction are very similar. The coffee drinker tends to drink coffee frequently, and some people drink up to eight cups of coffee or even more per day. In the long run, coffee is a nerve poison. Cola drinks, which contain much caffeine, are often the cause of the highly strung state of some children. Sleeplessness and depression are only some of the problems from which coffee drinkers suffer. Because coffee, like alcohol, stimulates kidney function and water elimination, it can really dry out the body.

Most children like chocolate drinks. Professor Mommsen, a well-known German paediatrician, wrote on this subject: 'Chocolate drinks often contain between 60 and 70 per cent sugar and, for this reason, should be rejected. These drinks also contain quite indigestible cacao, caffeine and saturated fats.'

Chocolate can provoke serious allergies, and when children eat or drink chocolate, they often lose their natural appetite. The biggest problem is that these drinks do not contain the natural complementary substances which would enable chocolate milk to be properly digested (the same applies to plain chocolate, which is a vitamin and mineral robber). However, these kinds of breakfast drinks sell very well and are very popular. Business always comes before health and its interests are sometimes even legally protected.

Most children prefer to ask for sweet drinks when they are thirsty. Although at first some of these drinks are thirst-quenching, after a short time the child again becomes thirsty, because of the sugar content in these drinks. Of course, this is the intention of the manufacturer. When thirsty, one should drink water – nothing but fresh, natural water.

How Much Should We Actually Drink?

'You ought to drink more! At least two litres per day!' Quite often we hear this well-meant advice. The general opinion that we should drink at least two litres per day stems from a very simple calculation.

On average, our body excretes daily about two and a half litres of liquid. Of course, one then assumes that this lost water has to be replaced. However, we forget that some foods contain much liquid. Some natural foods, like fruit, vegetables or rice, can consist of more than 90 per cent water.

What were things like in primeval times? Did people then make sure to drink at least two litres daily? Certainly not! In those times, they had no soft drinks or cola drinks, nor coffee or tea. Even water was not always available. But this was not as important as it seems, as those people lived exclusively on natural food which was full of water. Besides, in the tropical forests, there were many plants which contained liquid. Even today, there is a palm tree in the tropics which is called 'the travellers' palm tree'. Its leaves contain so much water that several people can drink sufficiently from it.

Animals such as rabbits, which eat 100 per cent raw food, drink hardly anything. The first primitive people did not eat any salt or sugar, with the possible exception of very small quantities of honey.

Our bodies can only process foods containing high concentrations of refined, unnatural substances when they have been diluted first. For this reason, we get thirsty when we eat such foods. Our brain regulates this process automatically. As nowadays we consume more and more of these indigestible foods, we are usually thirstier. Modern people have to drink plenty, otherwise they become dehydrated. We can no longer live like our ancestors.

How frequently one has to drink, and the amount of liquid one needs, is something very personal. It depends on how much we eat and what we eat, on our age and on several other factors. What is enough for one person may be insufficient for another. Somebody who eats in a way which nowadays is considered normal will need more liquid than a vegetarian who lives mainly on raw vegetables and eats little cooked food. The more salt or sugar and refined flour one eats, the more one needs to drink. Have you ever noticed that birds, when they eat bread, need lots of water? Athletes and people who do physical work and perspire a lot need more water than people who sit at their desks all day every day. In summer, we need more liquid than we do in the winter. When the weather is dry, we need more liquid than when it is humid.

As long as we are still young, we know when we are thirsty. The older we become, the less we notice when we ought to drink. Therefore, at a certain age, one has to be careful not to drink too little. We need at least one and a half litres per day. However, one should not drink just anything. Most modern drinks are not thirst-quenchers. We only drink these modern drinks to please our taste buds. Sometimes, as an exception to the rule, it is all right to enjoy an occasional cup of coffee or tea. But the only healthy drink is water, nothing but water. We should not overdo this either, though. We need water, but not in excessive quantities. It is said that water cleans and flushes the kidneys. This is true, but too much liquid puts stress on your kidneys and can have disastrous consequences. You should always keep to the happy medium and try to estimate yourself how much water on average you need per day.

NICOTINE

I grew up surrounded by the tobacco industry. My father made the finest cigars, which were well known all over the world. As a child, I often sat in the factory watching these cigars being made. When my father became aware that nicotine was an addictive substance, he left his job straight away, as his conscience would not permit him to stay in that trade. In my younger days, tobacco was much more socially acceptable, but if we look at tobacco today and what my father taught me about it, we see that it is an addiction that has cost many people their lives. About half of all regular cigarette smokers will eventually be killed by their habit.

In my daily treatment of patients, I see the struggle facing those who desperately want to stop smoking and who have bravely said, 'I'll stop it now.' Usually acupuncture is extremely successful, because it breaks the habit and breaks the desire. I also try to motivate those people struggling with their nicotine addiction by telling them what benefits they will get in return – better health, improved chest and lungs, enhanced taste and smell, and much more money in their pockets! I also tell them if they could see what a pathologist sees every day, they would stop immediately. Yet the spirit is willing but the flesh is weak – that is, until smoking hits them hard and their life is in danger. This is therefore another addiction that needs our careful consideration. If smokers had the ability to see inside their own bodies and look at what the habit is doing to their health, then they might stop. Simply telling them this, however, has no impact whatsoever. It is not until health problems crop up that the implications of years of inhaling cigarette smoke really hit them.

Smoking and Children's Health

Children can quickly become dependent on nicotine as a result of peer pressure to smoke. They become aware of cigarettes from an early age. By the age of eleven, one-third of children, and by sixteen two-thirds, have experimented with smoking. Children who experiment with cigarettes quickly become addicted to the nicotine in tobacco. Every year, between 80,000 and 100,000 children become addicted to tobacco worldwide. In the United Kingdom, about 450 children start smoking every day. In 1982, the first national survey of smoking among children found that 11 per cent of 11–16 year olds were smoking regularly. Almost a quarter of Britain's 15 year olds – both boys and girls – are regular smokers. Over half (58.5 per cent) of regular smokers aged between 11 and 15 years say that they would find it difficult to go without smoking for a week, while 72 per cent think they would find it difficult to give up altogether. During periods of abstinence, young people have withdrawal symptoms similar to those experienced by adult smokers.

Children are three times as likely to smoke if both of their parents smoke and parental approval or disapproval of the habit is also a significant factor. They are also influenced by their friends' and older siblings' smoking habits.

The earlier children become regular smokers, the greater their risk of dying prematurely if they persist in the habit as adults. A recent US study found that smoking during teenage years causes permanent changes in the lungs and increases the risk of developing lung cancer later in life, even if the smoker subsequently stops.

Children are also more susceptible to the effects of passive smoking. In households where both parents smoke, the children are, on average, receiving the equivalent in nicotine of smoking 80 cigarettes a year. Children of parents who smoke during the child's early life run a higher risk of cancer in adulthood, and the larger the number of smokers in a household, the greater the cancer risk to non-smokers in the family. Several hundred people die every year from lung cancer caused by passive smoking.

Parents who smoke cause between 8,000 and 26,000 new cases of childhood asthma in the US each year and exacerbate existing asthma in 20 per cent of the 2 to 5 million children who already have the disease. The saddest thing is that a survey reported that in the year 2000, 18 per cent of expectant mothers in England continued to smoke during pregnancy.

Smoking Prevention

Since the 1970s, health education about the effects of smoking has been included in the curricula of most primary and secondary schools in the UK, but this does not seem to affect smoking rates. Raising the cost of cigarettes can deter children from smoking. A recent American study has shown that while price does not appear to affect initial experimentation with smoking, it is an important tool in reducing youth smoking once the habit has become established.

The other day, I met a lady who stopped smoking two years ago following the treatment I administered, which included the use of acupuncture and some homoeopathic remedies. I felt so happy when she said, 'I have a new life. I have been on two cruises around the world since I stopped – paid for by the money I have saved since I gave up. For years, I polluted the air and my family and, for that, I feel very ashamed.'

I spend a lot of time offering support and guidance to young pregnant women who smoke, because I know what it is doing to their health and also to their babies. For those who manage to beat the habit, it is such a blessing. How satisfying it is to breathe in fresh air and not be in a constant fog of cigarette smoke. It is wonderful to be able to appreciate the clear, clean air that nature has given to us.

DRUGS

Whatever the drug is, whatever the craving is – be it cannabis, LSD, heroin, etc., or whether it is sweets, soft drinks, coffee, tea, chocolate, sedatives, painkillers, cigarettes, or other addictive substances – most people seem to need crutches in order to make their life bearable. These substances stimulate the 'reward' centre of the brain and, despite their varied nature, the pathways of the brain they affect are extremely similar.

In primeval times, cravings for sweets, starches and fats, as well as the chewing of certain relaxing herbs in times of danger, were needed for the survival of the human race. Now, the very same cravings have become addictions for millions of human beings, especially young people, who seem to need stronger and stronger substances and tranquillisers in order to survive. However, many new substances threaten to overpower and kill us instead of giving relief. The long-term use of alcohol or drugs can lead to changes in the brain structure. Addicted adolescents live in a perpetual haze and most of the time do not realise what they are doing. Without doubt, this is an important factor in the constantly growing crime rate.

Educational and health organisations have tried to halt this dangerous development, but most young people do not realise the danger and often couldn't care less. They do not worry about, say, getting lung cancer when they are old, reasoning that 'We've all got to die of something'. Teenagers have a strong belief in their own immortality – 'It won't happen to me.' For young people, it is hardly possible to estimate the personal risk. State and privately funded schools alike are overrun by the drug problem. It is rarely possible to catch a drug supplier without a tip-off and most pupils are far too scared to tell, for fear of violent retribution. Death threats are not uncommon.

British surveys suggest that 45 per cent of people aged 16–29 have used illegal drugs. It is estimated that 1.5 million ecstasy pills are taken every week in Britain. The Home Office reported that heroin addiction alone accounted for £1.3 billion in property crimes in 1997. One in five of all people arrested are heroin addicts.

As a consequence of bad living and eating habits and the lack of much-needed nutrients, many grown-ups suffer from biochemical deficiencies that are later inherited by their children. Our children are a mirror image of our industrial world. While destroying our soil, our water and our air, we are also destroying the health of our children. Children who are addicted to tobacco, alcohol and drugs cannot possibly recover without help, but all our measures to change the prevailing tendency towards self-destruction in our youth will be a waste of time, effort and money as long as we do not see the whole picture.

THESE PEOPLE NEED HELP – BUT HOW?

The most important thing is that the person in question really wants to get rid of their addiction. If the addiction has already become stronger than the desire for health, the addict will be unable to help themselves – they no longer care. Some people have found help with Alcoholics Anonymous (AA). If one becomes a member of this charitable organisation, one is no longer allowed to drink a single drop of alcohol. This is very difficult for most alcoholics, and only a few can keep it up. There is always the possibility of a relapse, even after many years. But this international organisation has achieved a lot of success and continues to do so. It should be viewed with great respect.

If they go into a clinic for detoxification, alcoholics are practically locked up for weeks and sometimes for months. Nobody there is allowed to drink alcohol and the common treatment consists of psychotherapy and pharmaceutical drugs, which often increase the lack of vital nutrients! After such a detoxification treatment and recovery, there are often relapses.

AA and most hospitals try to influence the addicted person's personality and behaviour. They want to change a weak character and strengthen the will-power. If people believe in God or another superior power, one tries to influence their wish to be abstinent through religious thoughts and prayers. Sometimes this works and people don't suffer a relapse.

Life is very hard for ex-alcoholics. Often they do not enjoy life any more because they live in fear of their own weakness. It is unbelievable how much distress and misery can be caused by treatments for addiction which attribute blame to the subject.

However, for many years, well-informed doctors and naturopaths have known that there are also other reasons for an addiction. An addiction can be caused by:

- an abnormal lack of certain vital nutrients (e.g. B vitamins)
- food allergies
- nutrition which lacks many vital substances
- food additives and junk food
- too many refined carbohydrates
- a weak immune system
- an environment containing many toxins
- great worries, anxiety and other personal problems

Most often, a combination of the various causes mentioned above triggers an addiction. Therefore it is important to have certain tests done. Among these are hair, blood and blood sugar tests, which should be done regularly in order to find out which deficiencies, allergies, toxins or other poisonous substances are involved. With the help of these tests, it will be possible to compose a very personal diet for each patient to supply them with the nutrients they lack. Every person who suffers from addiction should be treated in the same way as those who suffer from other diseases. The organism should first be cleaned and the further intake of harmful substances should be strictly avoided. Fasting is very important, and one should get into the habit of always eating as healthily as possible. Bowel movements should be regular and the bacterial flora should be sanitised. The intestines should be cleansed by enemas with camomile tea, and sometimes colon hydrotherapy can do miracles. Sufficient physical exercise and fresh air are very important.

The worst problem for the patient is total abstinence. To drink a glass of wine, not every day but now and then, can be very enjoyable. Even in ancient times, people liked to have a drink in order to relax. Yet this treat was always reserved for exceptional festive occasions. Providing the patient is not yet too addicted, total abstinence will only be necessary for a certain time, i.e. until there is no more lack of various vital substances, which can be proved by different tests. After this, they will be allowed to drink one or two glasses of wine occasionally, for example when there is a family party, but, especially in the beginning, their drinking habits will have to be strictly watched. Usually there will be no relapse if the person concerned always remembers to take a mixture of the substances they lack. There are specific nutrients which all alcoholics lack, while the intake of other substances would have to be tailored to the needs of each individual patient. As long as our 'civilisation food' is deficient in many ways, addictions will increase and the general health of the population will worsen.

The treatment detailed above is the only one which might really at last help some addicted persons and their relatives. Unfortunately, many doctors and nurses, and people with stubborn and dogmatic attitudes, will continue to ignore the facts mentioned above. It will be very difficult to change this kind of attitude as there is much ignorance, but eventually, common sense may again conquer dogmatism. Then, millions of people could be helped in a much better and more sensible way. If we want to experience health and happiness, then we have to look at the problems that rob us of these. Help is at hand. What is needed is a lot of common sense, perseverance and determination.

PREVENTING ADDICTION

Why is there such a demand for these addictive, health-endangering products? Why do our children need stimulants and tranquillisers? There are many different reasons, but most are closely related to the fact that many of our children are not really happy. They have a feeling of uselessness and of being lost. They do not understand their role; they see the futility of our modern way of life. Many parents cannot give them the stamina they need in order to withstand temptation and, on the contrary, often show them a bad example. The problems of our young people reflect those of our planet. As a result of modern agricultural techniques, our soil no longer has enough vitality to grow food full of the nutrients our children need. If we pollute our environment, we poison our children too.

Somewhere along the road real values have been lost and, in order to help our children, we must find them again. We are weak. We have lost our courage and will-power. We are watching our children drown, but we ourselves have never learnt to swim and we do not know how to save them. Hundreds of thousands of us join political marches: we want a different government, we want better leaders who will fight alcohol, tobacco and drugs and make life worthwhile and safe again. But what honest and honourable man wants to be a leader in our time, a leader of people who are weak and do not even have the courage to change their own lives; a leader of people who do not protest when their fields and farmlands, their water and the air they breathe are being poisoned for the sake of money and so-called progress; a leader of people who accept that once-wholesome food that in the past served to build a healthy and courageous people is being exchanged for artificial products that would be inedible without many thousands of additives, colourings and taste-enhancers; a leader of people who accept that their children have become alcoholics and drug addicts, without trying to give up their own bad habits? Most people have lost belief in themselves; they are weak, even weaker than their own children, who are the real victims.

Of course, there are still some people who try to fight, to do the right things, but they are only a small minority, and most people nowadays are of the opinion that it is better to do nothing at all than take a risk. Millions of us go to church every Sunday, but during the week we forget the promises we made and do nothing while watching our children suffer.

When I was young, we ate simple and wholesome food, and we still knew how to be happy and play games. Most modern children do not know how to play simple games any more. They are used to video games where winning, shooting, killing and the subjection of others to violence are of the greatest importance. Modern children need these games, however, in order to know how to defend themselves in real life.

For our young children, we buy noisy toys that can harm their hearing beyond repair. When these children grow up, they need even more noise in order to get a feeling of being unimpeachable and strong. The weaker their personality and the more hopeless and downtrodden teenagers feel, the more noise they will make to regain some of their lost self-assurance.

Many children, especially those living in towns, do not know the wonderful feelings of happiness and peace one can find in natural surroundings. They do not know any more how to daydream while listening to the song of birds or watching the clouds. They do not know that all living things – plants, animals and human beings – have their own special place in the world. Nature is the best teacher. As soon as children have the opportunity to observe nature by themselves, they will be able to understand it and, by and by, they will lose their feelings of loneliness and incompetence.

Everything living in the world has its own very special assignment. Every human being, every child, has a unique personality and special talents that nobody else has. All life is interlocked, and all forms of life need one another. Everyone is responsible for the health and welfare of all children. The only way to get out of the spiral of addiction, towards a free and happy life, is to start, not tomorrow but today, to change our own lives and save the children who can still be saved.

Most children don't know the joy of living any more. Start by giving your children more care, more fun and, above all, more love and understanding. Do things together with your children – hiking and camping, or sailing and rowing. Let them know that you need them, and show them nature, birds and flowers. Explain to them that all human beings are responsible for their own lives. Teach them the value of healthy food and a healthy lifestyle, and never say no without explaining why. Shake yourself up – drink less alcohol and coffee and fewer soft drinks, eat fewer sweets and less junk food, stop smoking and try to show your children in everything you do that you are fighting your own bad habits, because happiness is worth fighting for. Your head will become clear again and life will be much happier. Your example is the most important thing for your children. They will be proud of you and will learn to be proud of themselves.

I once read: 'The greatest phase in man's advancement is that in which he passes from subconscious to conscious control of his own mind and body.' This saying has become my favourite quotation. No human is born to be a slave, either to other people or to their own weaknesses. Everyone has the inborn material for further development and greatness, and should learn to use what is given to them so that they can be proud and happy.

The first thing young people must learn is to have the courage to stand up and resist the influence of others in their life. They should be honest with themselves and live according to their own beliefs about what is right and wrong for them. I would love to tell all young people, 'Jump from the bandwagon and start the adventure of living your own life. Escape while there still is time and you still have the will-power to do it. It will not always be easy, you will have to learn much and work hard until you are really independent, but you can do it. Anything is better than being the chattel and slave of some self-appointed leader, being his or her dependent and feeble-minded groupie. Take the road of real happiness, from the slavery of addiction towards freedom.'

When we look at all these addictive substances, it is almost unbelievable to comprehend that sugar might be just as addictive as heroin. They are, nonetheless, all addictions that we should be able to control. The stresses and strains of modern-day life can play a part in these addictions, so it is important that we learn how to relax in order to overcome them. The following method, which has been practised through the ages, is often very successful. It is a healing treatment that should be carried out regularly by a trained practitioner in order for it to work.

One has to realise that there are billions of cells in a square inch of tissue in the human body. These cells have intelligence; they take in oxygen plus the necessary elements they require to sustain them; they breathe and excrete waste matter. They can live independently of the rest of the body and – a most important factor – indefinitely when placed in a suitable nutrient solution. This is a scientific fact.

The thought forms of love, sympathy and compassion – being of a positive nature – neutralise and restore the rhythmic balance of diseased cells. Many schools of thought and therapeutics stress the point that man has within him the means to heal himself.

It is very simple – when emotions such as worry, fear, anxiety, jealousy, hatred, anger, revenge, even timidity and bashfulness develop in our minds, they will short-circuit the flow of magnetic energy to and from the organs of the body via the spinal cord. Where they break and pass each other, an eddy of magnetism is set up. There is no medicine or instrument that will cause these vortices to cease. These are a form of trigger spot.

Seven places down the neck and spine need to be contacted magnetically to eliminate all these triggers. Three of the worst are located in the neck, three more are found just below the neck (between the shoulder blades and on down the spine) and the last one is located far down the spine in the region of the hips.

The positive half of any treatment is given with the right hand applied to the left side of the afflicted person. The negative half is given by the left hand on the right side of the spine. In reality, only the thumbs are used – right thumb on left side and left thumb on right side. Before beginning, the practitioner should close the hands (just gently), so that the energy of the fingers will flow back into the palms. During the treatment, the thumbs should never be placed directly on top of the vertebrae, but rather alongside them. You will notice that, down the neck and back, the vertebrae protrude upward in a long row. On each side of these there is a depression. It is in this low place, alongside the points of the vertebrae, that the thumbs are placed for either a positive or negative treatment. These grooves are about an inch away from the spine and affect the sympathetic nervous system. The therapist should never apply any pressure when giving a magnetic treatment. A light, even, steady contact with the balls of the thumbs on each side is all that is needed to allow the release of the triggers. Each application of the thumbs will last for about two minutes. The practitioner should take a deep breath before each application and then breathe normally.

The first place where we normalise magnetically is located down the neck, just a little distance below the skull (axis).

The second place is just halfway down the neck (third to fourth cervical).

The third is at the base of the neck (seventh cervical).

The fourth is just about an inch below the third place and is in the region of the first dorsal vertebra.

The fifth place is in the vicinity of the third dorsal.

The sixth is at the fifth dorsal.

The seventh is at the base of the spine in the region of the third lumbar.

This treatment will not only bring a healing force to the body but will also boost one's determination to succeed in fighting addiction.

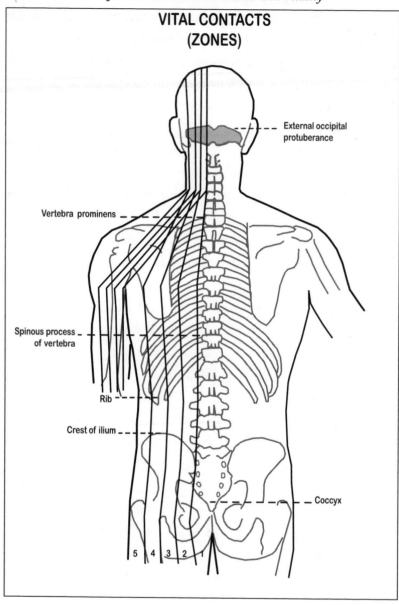

The zones contacted in magnetic treatment

There are many ways in which one can help oneself, and in my books *Stress and Nervous Disorders* and *Inner Harmony,* you will find a lot of ways to help solve the problems of stress and addiction and, for those who are suffering, hopefully these will bring about success.

CHAPTER FOUR

Natural Ways to Keep Skin, Hair and Nails Healthy

SKIN

It was a long time ago that Cleopatra bathed in ass's milk to keep her skin soft and beautiful, but to this day, everyone would like to be able to retain their youthful looks and to keep healthy for as long as possible. It is not just women who pride themselves on having fresh-looking skin, silky hair and strong nails, but men too pay great attention to their grooming and appearance.

The body is covered entirely with skin from top to toe. The skin is, in fact, a very complex organ and has a totally different role from, for example, the skin of a cheese. A person's skin is responsible for many different functions. It is a mighty weapon, acting as a barrier against outside influences, and has a vitally important role in maintaining a constant body temperature of 37°C. The skin also behaves like a third kidney: in controlling perspiration, for example, it filters out waste products and ensures that we do not dehydrate.

The skin is one of the biggest organs of the body and a man has roughly 1.5 sq. m. of skin, weighing about 4.5 kg, with 10 kg of fat underneath. The skin of a female, on the other hand, weighs about 3 kg and the fat underneath weighs 12 kg.

Skin is made up of two layers – the outer (or superficial) layer is called the epidermis, while the deeper layer is known as the dermis. Depending on what is required from the skin, it can be thick and rough or fine and supple. Hormonal secretions determine whether the skin is dry or oily. All over the body, with the exception of the lips, the skin is covered with sweat glands. There are about three million sweat glands, mostly on the palms of the hands and the soles of the feet, and also in the armpits. These allow perspiration to maintain the body temperature although, especially under the armpits, perspiration can often result in an unpleasant odour and is also a common cause of many skin conditions.

I have just touched briefly on the functions of the skin here. As I have already covered skin disorders in my book *Skin Diseases,* I want in this chapter to focus on how to keep the skin, hair and nails healthy.

The Sebaceous Glands

The sebaceous glands have an important part to play. Alfred Vogel, my business partner, recorded some very important facts about these and believed that these glands are as important as the sweat glands.

Our skin is like living leather, with a built-in, automatic lubrication system, in the form of the sebaceous glands, that becomes active in accordance with the skin's needs. Dry skin (lacking oil) is extremely sensitive, making one much more susceptible to colds and infections, and also to radiation damage. Washing with soap not only removes dirt but also causes sebum, the lubricant secreted by the sebaceous glands, to be dissolved at the same time. This means that the skin is deprived of the necessary oil, and its protective function is diminished. For this reason, it is especially important in the winter to use a good skin oil after washing with soap. Experience has shown that St John's wort oil is the best skincare oil known to us. It is truly excellent for the skin and especially for the capillaries and nerves embedded in it. However, since it is rather greasy, it should be mixed with essential oils from plants, which provide the added bonus of enhancing the soothing effect of the St John's wort oil. It would be a good idea to keep a bottle in your bathroom on account of its importance in skincare and as a massage oil.

If there is insufficient secretion from the sebaceous glands, causing the skin to be rough and chapped, the application of a cream containing lanolin is required. *Chamomile Ointment* is a natural and effective remedial cream that is soon able to revitalise the skin. This tried and tested cream contains lanolin as a base, as well as arnica, sanicle and other medicinal herbs that have proved their worth in skincare. *Chamomile Ointment* is also recommended as a protection against sunburn, with the best results being obtained if it is applied to the skin the day before exposure to the sun.

The Sweat Glands

The manifold functions of the sweat glands have only gradually come to be recognised. The body has about two million sweat glands, each one being about five millimetres (about one-fifth of an inch) long. Even without perspiring, they evaporate 1–1.5 litres (1.7–2.6 pints) of water during the course of a day. If exudation is increased by means of a steam bath or sauna or as a result of living in the tropics, the body is able to produce up to ten times this quantity of water.

If it were possible to combine all the pores into one single tube, its diameter would be about 25–30 cm (10–12 inches). The size of such a tube makes it easy to understand why so much liquid is able to escape. Taste a drop of sweat and you will find that it is salty. On litmus paper its reaction is acid. In fact, sweat contains sodium salts, potassium, sulphuric acid, iron, phosphorus, lactic acid and as much urea as one kidney excretes, which is why the skin could be called the 'third kidney'. The skin can exude arsenic and other poisons, sometimes resulting in eczema and other skin eruptions. This shows the wisdom of treating skin problems internally as well as externally. Indeed, it explains why sweat treatments have cured many an illness.

The sweat glands are the units of a temperature-control system that makes life in hot countries more bearable. By evaporating water through the sweat glands, it is possible to lose heat of up to 500 calories. Keep the skin in good working order and you will be observing one of the most important rules for good health.

When Alfred Vogel visited Mesopotamia (between the Euphrates and Tigris rivers), he went to a small museum at the edge of the ruined city of ancient Babylon. There he saw vessels that had been used by women of those bygone times for the storage of oils and creams. According to ancient records, the women used plants as a basis for the preparation of cosmetics and aromatic oils, as is still the practice among Arab and Bedouin women in those areas. On another visit, this time to the Indians of the Amazon region, he became acquainted with a plant from which a fatty red dye is obtained. The natives use this extract to paint the body and face, and it adheres to the skin for weeks, not even soap being strong enough to remove it.

Beauty culture is almost as old as the human race. The desire to look attractive and to improve one's looks is somehow inborn, and it is women especially who take full advantage of the possibilities. However, although cosmetics can be beneficial to the skin and its functions, they can also be detrimental, as are all creams and other preparations that block the pores and impair or completely stop the exudation of sweat, thus making the skin flaccid and tired looking. Frequent powdering also has the same effect. This explains why some women certainly do not look their best without their make-up and can give you quite a shock if you see them first thing in the morning. Without make-up, a 40-year-old woman who has been accustomed to applying non-biological cosmetics for many years may look like a 70-year-old grandmother.

The skin can and should be the expression of one's good health, so if you want to help nature a little by caring for your skin, use nothing but biological cosmetics, especially those of natural plant origin, since they stimulate and support the skin's natural functions. Other cosmetics are little more than paint, a veritable deception.

When the Functions of the Skin are Impaired

It is understandable that tribal peoples in, for example, Africa, South America and the South Sea Islands enjoy a better skin function than people who have to wear thick clothing all the time. Tribes such as the Amazonian Jivaro often walk around wearing very little clothing, if any, and their bodies are in constant contact with the air, with sunlight and often with muddy water, thus promoting a more efficient skin function. Since in colder regions of the earth it would be impossible to do this, the people living in northern Europe must have followed a healthy, instinctive desire to stimulate their bodies by taking regular saunas and improving the effect even further by cooling down afterwards in cold water or by rolling in the snow, for these customs also keep the functions of the skin in good order and, in turn, benefit the whole body.

For the same reason, some people with a healthy instinct like to go hiking or swimming. They practise such a sport on a reasonable scale, and if they ski, it is done in a sensible way, climbing up the mountain slope instead of using a ski lift. Other people find greater pleasure and benefit in massaging the body or having it massaged regularly. They use an effective oil that stimulates the functions of the skin, keeping it healthy and in top condition.

Impaired skin functions can have extremely detrimental

consequences. If you do not perspire enough, you should frequently drink an infusion of elderflower, peppermint and lovage – you can take them either in alternation or as a mixed herb tea. In addition, it is recommended that you take a sauna weekly over an extended period.

Certain parts of the body can sweat excessively, for example the hands, feet and armpits. Is there anything one can do about this condition? Yes, there is. You can stimulate the kidneys with a good kidney tea containing *Solidago* (goldenrod) or by taking *A. Vogel Solidago Complex.* The skin, the so-called third kidney, will be relieved as soon as the kidneys themselves have been activated. Additionally, in accordance with the methods of the ancient Chinese, take sage tea or *Salvia* drops (made from fresh sage) regularly. If the perspiration, especially under the arms, has an unpleasant smell, the best external remedy is *Hamamelis* soap, which contains witch hazel and thyme, and is an excellent means of supporting the treatment with sage drops or tea. Washing daily with *Hamamelis* soap, followed by the application of *Chamomile Ointment* has also proved successful in cases of feet that sweat excessively.

In a recent broadcast, I was asked several questions on how to alleviate blushing and perspiration covering the whole body. I was surprised at the huge response I had from that programme, following which I was able to help a great number of people by prescribing *Solidago Complex* (15 drops to be taken twice daily) and *Golden Grass Tea* which are both advisable for these conditions. Those who are bothered by these symptoms should also study their diet and particularly try to eliminate salt and spicy foods as much as possible.

Dry, scaly skin that is flaking off can be effectively treated by the external application of St John's wort oil in alternation with *Comfrey Cream* or *Symphosan,* which contain comfrey and other herbs. At the same time, take *Viola tricolor,* a tincture made from heartsease (wild pansy). If the condition is caused by dry psoriasis, you will also have to dab the affected area with *Molkosan* every day. Calluses, skin that is hard as a lizard's, are the result of a disease of the endocrine glands, often connected with avitaminosis (a disease caused by vitamin deficiency), and will require special treatment of the underlying cause.

Skin Blemishes

No one likes to have skin blemishes, but it is not uncommon for young people to have a problem with spots, especially during puberty. A spotty face can even create an inferiority complex if all lotions and creams fail to help. This is another reason why the problem of impure skin should be tackled at the roots. The recommendation to be careful about what one eats and adopt an appropriate diet is not always received with appreciation, but it is necessary, since the trouble is basically the result of ingesting the wrong food.

If you suffer from spots, it is of the utmost importance that you reduce your intake of fats by half or three-quarters. What is more, take great care to avoid fats and oils which have been heated, animal fats being especially detrimental. Cakes, biscuits, pastries and all other sweets should be left out of the diet altogether or at least drastically reduced. Eggs, particularly boiled eggs, omelettes and other hot egg dishes are like poison for impure skin. Only fresh soft white cheeses, such as cottage cheese or quark, are digestible; no other kind of cheese should be eaten. Raw vegetables, natural brown rice, potatoes boiled in their skins, cottage cheese and horseradish are nutritive and remedial, and contain plenty of essential vitamins and minerals. Hot spices tend to make things worse.

Some external remedies that have proved very effective are *Echinaforce* and *Molkosan* – one day apply *Echinaforce* to the affected area, the next day use *Molkosan* and continue in daily alternation. Apply a little *Chamomile Ointment* to any patches of dry skin. For internal treatment, take *Viola tricolor* and also *Echinaforce*.

Avoid squeezing spots and blackheads, unless you apply *Molkosan* to disinfect them right away, otherwise you will only spread the bacteria, which usually settles in the inflamed skin pores. In other words, if you want to prevent the condition from getting worse, you have to be very careful. Also, do not handle or work with turpentine, floor wax, paints and modern detergents. If you have to use them, make sure you wear rubber gloves for protection. And another thing: it is not always advisable to wash with soap. Cleansing the skin with oil and then wiping it with alcohol is often more beneficial for impure skin.

A range of products I have formulated, which are totally herb-based, give tremendous results with the most troublesome skin problems. Natural remedies like *AcneZyme* and *Skin Factors* can improve conditions such as acne vulgaris and acne rosacea greatly. Blemishes of the skin can also be helped tremendously by the use of electro-acupuncture. This treatment is also beneficial to those who have been maimed in accidents or in fires. It is really quite amazing what can be done to improve difficult situations.

Finally, I cannot emphasise strongly enough how important it is to improve your general health by adopting a natural way of life. Your skin will then derive great benefits too.

Should Oils be Used for Skincare?

It is true that nature itself sees to it that our skin receives the oil it needs, and for this purpose we have been given the marvellous sebaceous glands, which work automatically. I have noticed that people in less developed parts of the world tend to have much oilier skin than we have and they never have to worry about dry skin. Unfortunately, the sebaceous glands of people living in industrialised societies work less efficiently and there is a very good reason for this. The fact that we go against rather than cooperate with nature – through our unnatural way of life, our food, clothing and general living conditions, and doing our work shut inside closed rooms that are often overheated in cold weather – discourages the proper functioning of the skin and the sebaceous glands.

To remedy this situation, we must give our skin all the help it needs in the form of a good oil. It is advisable to always lubricate the body well before going for a swim, whether in a cool freshwater lake or river or in the sea. Doing this will help the body to retain its warmth and you will not shiver or feel chilled, even if the water is cold. I am writing this from personal experience, although I must admit that I have a good basal metabolic rate and circulation, so I do not chill easily. The oil treatment is especially recommended for sensitive people, even more so for the prevention of chills after stepping out of the water.

On the other hand, it is not necessary and does not benefit the skin in any way to smear so much oil on the body that it looks greasy. Oil should be used sparingly and massaged well into the skin. Avoid oils that are scented with synthetic perfumes which can be smelled even from a distance. Pure olive oil mixed with a little lemon oil is a good and inexpensive skin lotion for bathing. If you want to buy a ready-made oil, look for a skin oil that is based on St John's wort oil, because this is a most excellent skin food on account of the lipoids it contains. It is important when shopping for this to ask for a skin oil that is made from natural, red St John's wort oil – reject any oil that is artificially coloured.

Care of the skin requires not only the use of oil but also common sense when exposing the body to the sun, light and air. An efficient skin function is the basis for proper glandular function and for general well-being.

Wrinkles and Skin with Large Pores

As a rule, smooth skin is a sign of youthfulness and good health, and it is not surprising that women in particular make a great effort to maintain this desirable condition for as long as they possibly can. But it is not simply a matter of giving nature a helping hand by applying plenty of powder, make-up and creams. In fact, the liberal use of such products may achieve just the opposite of what is desired. The real answer lies in taking care in one's youth, living in a natural way and not worrying too much or constantly giving in to anxieties, for we know that stress is wearisome and undermines the body's reserves and well-being. It does indeed age us prematurely and fosters the formation of wrinkles. Of course, constant tiredness on account of overwork or pursuing pleasure night after night can also harm one's health and impair one's youthful looks. It is understandable that so many people want to cover up these flaws on their faces by using all kinds of cosmetics.

What is less understandable is why some girls plaster their young and radiant faces with make-up. Make-up is supposed to hide what is ugly, but what could be more beautiful than glowing health, smooth and youthful skin, red cheeks and lips as nature coloured them?

The skin cannot breathe naturally if the pores are blocked with cosmetics. In consequence, it degenerates – the pores become larger. It is just as unsightly when the skin begins to slacken early, developing more wrinkles than would be expected as a result of the normal ageing process.

Many ladies come to me with skin problems, particularly with concerns about lines, crow's feet and wrinkles. In such cases, I usually carry out a course of electro-acupuncture, which can prove very effective. For those with large pores, I would prescribe *Comfrey Cream*, which does a wonderful job.

Sensible, Natural Skincare

It is important that the skincare you practise protects and benefits the skin rather than damaging it. The reason why I raise this point is the great number of cosmetics on the market and the persuasive advertising used to sell them. Unfortunately, only very few of this host of products really are kind to the skin. You see, the term 'skincare' only applies correctly to products that protect the skin, are good for it, keep it healthy, indeed even heal and rejuvenate it. Only skin that functions properly can remain healthy and reflect freshness, perhaps even youthfulness. This requires first and foremost good circulation, for without this adequate nourishment for the skin is impossible.

Much time is often wasted in efforts to improve the looks with cosmetics. Yet how much easier it would be to keep the body healthy and, in particular, to take good care of the sex glands right from the start. Their efficiency contributes to maintaining youthfulness longer. For this, sunlight, deep-breathing and exercise are important. Anyone who spends most of their time in heated rooms, rarely moves around in the open air, never goes for walks or hikes or practises some other sport in moderation should not be surprised if they become like a hothouse plant and grow old before their time. Remember, exercise in the open air, perhaps gardening or walking, has much to do with keeping young and fit. Regular showers alternating between hot and cold water are also beneficial since they promote good circulation.

Another factor to consider is the importance of stimulating the skin's ability to breathe, or at least ensuring that this is not impaired. Cosmetics that block the pores prevent the skin from breathing properly. Such products include powder, certain other cosmetics and many creams containing fat, filling materials and stabilisers which the skin is unable to absorb. If the skin is not treated in the right way, it will begin to look withered and will age prematurely.

In addition to physical treatment to stimulate the circulation and regenerate the skin, there are some first-class plants that can be used for this purpose. St John's wort (*Hypericum*) is most frequently indicated and widely used. Its oil-soluble ingredients promote good circulation in the skin because even the finest capillaries will be activated. Plants that contain mucilage, for example comfrey and some mosses, rejuvenate the skin and, in time, can even soften wrinkles, since the skin tissue will recover its youthful tone. It is therefore most beneficial in the care of your face if you soak some cotton wool with *Symphosan* and dab your face with it after washing, or regularly apply *Comfrey Cream*. Should you suffer from eczema and dry skin, wash the affected areas with an infusion of heartsease (wild pansy) every day.

Badly functioning sebaceous glands tend to dry the skin and require the use of a cream made from plant oils, lanolin and vitamin F. Whatever cream you decide on, it should supply the skin with the substances it lacks. Creams with a Vaseline base are not truly satisfactory because Vaseline is difficult to saponify and the skin cannot absorb it. *Chamomile Ointment,* on the other hand, is excellent for dry, even cracked and chapped, skin. I would advise that any rich skin cream be applied sparingly. Remember, too, that the skin absorbs oil or fat more quickly in cold weather than in warm weather.

Non-greasy creams based on something other than plant mucilage generally contain ingredients that block the pores. The skin suffers and loses its smoothness if the treatment continues for some time. Oiling the skin, especially after washing with soap, is to be recommended, since soap removes the natural oil produced by the sebaceous glands. A good oil that stimulates the skin is indispensable in winter and whenever engaging in water sports.

It is imperative that the perfumes added to skin oils and creams come only from natural essential oils. Perfumes derived from chemicals can harm the skin. Also, remember that the skin derives no benefit whatsoever from being covered with thick layers of all kinds of cosmetics. Healthy skin only needs a little help when greater demands than usual are put on it through exposure to the sun, water, cold or wind. The wisdom expressed in the saying 'You can have too much of a good thing', applies to the care of your skin and to cosmetics too.

For a basic, reliable skincare programme, rub in *Comfrey Cream* every morning after washing. Afterwards, as a protection against strong sunlight or biting wind (it is not necessary to do this daily), apply *Chamomile Ointment,* which contains lanolin. Then, before going to bed, soak a cotton pad with *Viola tricolor* and dab over the whole face. In order to help the sebaceous glands, use a natural skin oil, or the lanolin cream already mentioned, two or three times a week. This regime will be sufficient for everyday use, provided you are not generally exposed to cold and sunshine. It is quite a simple treatment and you will derive great benefits if you take care of your skin like this for a few months. It will look much younger and the pores will be reduced in size.

So much can be done to help improve skin complaints. Young girls are very conscious of imperfections in their skin and often come to me pleading, 'Please help me to get rid of these nasty pimples.' In these instances, there is so much that can be done with the remedies that I have already mentioned together with a thorough skincare programme.

NAILS

The appearance of the hands is very important; they are one of the first things that people notice about you when you meet. Most people are particularly conscious of their nails if they do not look attractive, whether it be something minor like a broken nail or a more serious fungal infection.

Diseases of the Nails

It is one of nature's wonders that the body is able to use silica and other minerals to provide the toes and fingers with tough, horny plates. By diseases of the nails, I do not mean deformities of the nails and diseases of the nail roots caused by the use of nail polish, manicures, etc. The nails and hair are usually an indication of the person's general condition of health. As a rule, those who suffer from metabolic disorders have neither strong nails nor healthy-looking hair. The nails and hair become brittle and lose their natural structure when there is a deficiency of minerals and trace elements. In such cases, the only worthwhile thing to do is to treat the basic cause of the problem. Eating food that is rich in calcium and silica is an excellent way to strengthen the nails, as is the supplementary intake of *A. Vogel Urticalcin* and *Galeopsis*.

Fungal nail infections are very common nowadays and lots of people contact me about the state of their nails when they have acquired such a problem. One has to be very careful, as the structure of the nails is important. No matter what fungal infection occurs or where, it is difficult to eradicate. However, as with all skin conditions, whey has proved to be of excellent value even for mycotic diseases, that is, fungal skin diseases. But since not everyone is able to go to a dairy in the country and obtain fresh whey, many patients like to use the concentrated whey as available in *Molkosan*.

A patient told me once that she had suffered from this troublesome problem for years, despite all her efforts to get rid of it. The fungus had settled under her breasts and on her arms, causing frequent soreness, and for more than 12 years she had used all kinds of remedies without success. Then she learned about *Molkosan* and an African plant remedy, *Spilanthes,* which complements and reinforces the healing effect of *Molkosan*. After applying these two remedies in alternation for about two weeks, she was pleased to note great improvement. The skin had been rehabilitated and was clear once again.

It goes without saying that such a splendid result makes one glad, if only because of the great patience the sufferer must have had in order to endure the unpleasant problem and its bothersome effects during years of unsuccessful treatment. Think of the discouragement and disappointment first of all, then the great relief when the stubborn fungus disappeared in a relatively short space of time, the skin restored to normal.

Athlete's foot and nail mycosis are stubborn infections. It is easy to acquire the fungus from infected scales of skin dropped on the floor of changing rooms in public swimming baths, or through contact with persons who suffer from the infection. If you want to treat these infections successfully, you will have to cut the nails to the quick, perhaps even using a nail file. Apply *Chamomile Ointment* during the day, and before you go to bed tie some absorbent cotton soaked in *Molkosan* round the affected areas, leaving it on all night. The following night, *Spilanthes* should be used instead of *Molkosan*. Continue applying these two remedies in alternation for quite some time. I remember one doctor from Berlin telling me quite excitedly that in his many years of medical practice, he had never known an effective remedy for athlete's foot and nail mycosis until, by chance, he came across *Molkosan* whey concentrate when he was standing in for another doctor elsewhere. The good results achieved in combating these infections may be due to the effect of concentrated lactic acid together with lactic enzymes and nutritive salts.

A simple inflammation of the cuticle can be treated successfully with *Chamomile Ointment, Molkosan* and *Echinaforce*. For the treatment of more serious cases of inflammation, for example onychia, use horseradish tincture instead of *Molkosan*. The use of *Urticalcin* is generally very beneficial, as is *Silicea* (one teaspoonful taken twice daily). For external use, try *Propolis N* or, when warts or hard skin are present, then *Propolis H* will be very helpful in keeping nails strong and as healthy as possible.

HAIR

This brings us to an even more important part, which is the crowning glory of the head – our hair. There is nothing nicer for men and women to have than a healthy head of hair. Unfortunately, this can easily be disturbed. When I worked in India, they had an old saying, 'If there is baldness towards the front, it has an atmospheric cause; if the baldness is on the top, it is hormonal; if it affects the back of the head, then it is genetic; but when it comes out in patches, then there is usually an infection.'

I see lots of people nowadays with hair problems. I often find these to be caused by inefficient liver function or by a lack of keratin. In either case, the deficiency needs to be dealt with. There are some brilliant remedies available, such as *Hair, Skin and Nails* by Michael's (one tablet taken twice daily) or, to thoroughly cleanse the liver, *Detox Box* or *Milk Thistle Complex* – both by A. Vogel/Bioforce – can really work wonders.

Alfred Vogel said something worth remembering: 'Beautiful hair is a natural adornment.' Visitors to oriental countries cannot help but notice the many, mainly young, Buddhist monks clad in orange robes and with their heads shaved. They are to be seen everywhere. Without even thinking, you will compare them to the ordinary people with their beautiful dark hair. You will be convinced that hair is indeed an adornment. Women with auburn hair were considered especially beautiful in ancient Greece. But when we look at the thick bluish-black hair of indigenous peoples in the Americas and India, we may feel admiration or even a little envy – their bountiful hair is so desirable. These people do not yet have any need to spend money on preserving their beautiful locks. Baldness must be an acquired characteristic; it simply cannot have been the Creator's original intention – it is presumably a consequence of civilisation.

The Structure of the Hair

The anatomic structure of the hair, like so many other things in the body, is a technical miracle. Although the hair has no feeling, it is not dead matter either. Perhaps it could best be compared to a plant with a bulb-shaped root. The hair root, or bulb, is embedded in the skin, about three to five millimetres (an eighth to a fifth of an inch) deep, and is connected to blood vessels from which it receives the nutrients necessary for the hair to grow. The daily rate of growth is about a quarter to half a millimetre. A tightly knit network of lymphatics envelops the hair roots. The salty lymph is thought to act as an electrolyte in the electrical function of hair. Strong electric charges in hair can cause visible sparks when it is combed in the dark. The hair of very excited or ecstatic people lights up in the dark and, when photographed, this can be seen as a kind of halo. The effects of great mental disturbance and agitation are observable in the hair when viewed under a microscope, as notches of variable depths. So it is possible, for example, to discover if someone has had a nervous breakdown in the previous year by looking at their hair.

A medical book I once read described hair as the 'barometer of the soul'. In fact, extreme shock can make one's hair turn grey in a short time. People who have been buried under rubble when conscious and only freed some days later have been known to emerge grey-haired. When Alfred Vogel visited a hospital in Guatemala, he observed Indian children whose long black hair showed strains of white, in this case caused by vitamin deficiencies. Their bodies had lost the ability to produce black pigment the moment the deficiency disease started and the colour of the hair remained white as long as the disease lasted. Only after recovery did the hair return to its original black.

We can see, then, that the hair not only mirrors what goes on in our mind, but also our physical condition. For instance, during pregnancy, some women's hair becomes very oily due to increased activity of the sebaceous glands, but once the child is born, the function of the glands returns to normal, and with it the condition of the hair. The same principle applies in the case of animals. A shiny coat in dogs and horses is a sign of good health, but if it is dull or rough-looking, it is high time that the vet had a look to try and discover the underlying problem in the animal's system.

A healthy hair is strong, being able to support a weight of about 80 g (just under 3 oz) without snapping. A diseased hair, however, will tear when a weight of 30–40 g (about 1½ oz) is suspended from it. The healthy pigtail of a Chinese or Indian woman is able to support about 2½–3 tons before it snaps. Of course, the resistance of a single hair depends also upon its relative thickness. People who live close to nature have thicker and stronger hair than those who do not. Generally speaking, the more refined our food and lifestyle, the finer will be our hair.

When a hair is pulled out, the root, held fast in the dermis, is able to manufacture another hair shaft. However, eczema and other diseases affecting the scalp can cause this part to degenerate and die, so that the affected areas become bald. Typhoid fever usually results in the loss of all hair, but the hair bulb does not actually die, and the hair has been known to grow back even more luxuriantly after recovery when the capillary vessels and lymphatics have returned to their normal functions.

Hair Colour

The colour of the hair is manufactured near the roots, where an inner layer of cells contains pigments of various colours. That is why there are so many shades of hair, from blond to red to black. Hair colour is part of an individual's genetic make-up. True, the hairdresser can use chemicals to change your natural shade to one that is completely different. Nevertheless, the original colour will return at the roots as the hair continues to grow. So, if your hair is dyed or bleached and you do not wish it to be known, you will have to see your hairdresser regularly for a touch-up.

It has become the fashion to change one's hair colour according to a whim, but this may not always be appreciated by the passport control at international borders, for example, unless you have the 'hair colour' entry on your passport altered accordingly. Irrespective of modern extremes and changes, the natural variety of hair colours and characteristics is just as lovely as the charming variety of shape and colour seen in butterflies, birds, fish and other marine creatures, not forgetting the beauty of flowers.

Turning grey seems to be somehow connected with the activity of the sex glands. The hormone production of these glands diminishes with advancing age and the hair seems to go grey at the same rate. As already mentioned, however, dramatic mental and emotional shock, as well as continual stress and worries, can also be responsible for premature greying. It is often noticeable that during periods of stress the activity of the gonads is weakened. It may be down to genetics that some people turn grey in the bloom of youth. Unfortunately, however, grey hair does not usually suit the person's youthful looks. It is different with a face wrinkled as a result of rich experience and a hard life – silver-grey hair in such a person often seems a fitting crown.

Care of the Hair

Natural beauty calls for care if it is to remain, and this principle applies to our hair too. The best care we can give it is a natural way of life with plenty of exercise in the open air and a sensible diet. Remember, the hair is a reflection of our general condition of health. Most people look after their hair in one way or another, even though they may not have grasped the idea that the basic care and treatment has to be from inside the body itself. In other words, by eliminating any existing internal deficiencies, the appearance of the hair will improve. I often hear from patients who have taken silica and a biological calcium preparation who tell me, 'My hair is beautiful again.' They are elated and surprised at the same time.

Some older men try to keep their hair by using expensive tonics, but these preparations often benefit the manufacturers and advertisers more than those who would like to cure to their baldness. Really, all is in vain, because once the hair bulbs have gone, no new hair can grow. External care will no doubt benefit your hair to some extent. If, however, you do not see to it that you put your 'internal house' (your body) in order and do not take in sufficient calcium and silica, all external treatments will be of little use. It is really quite easy to do something about it.

Since hair contains silica, iron, copper, arsenic, manganese and sulphur, it stands to reason that plants in which these elements are found prove to be excellent for its care. People with naturally blond hair will find that washing their hair with camomile and then applying onion hair tonic is a superb treatment. Dark-haired people achieve better results with birch or nettle lotions. If you rinse your hair with diluted *Molkosan* (3 tablespoons to 1 litre/1¾ pints of water), it will retain its natural brilliance.

For care of the scalp and to combat hair loss, massage it with *Chamomile Ointment,* preferably a day before washing it. This natural cream contains lanolin, St John's wort oil and extracts of fresh plants. If fungal disease has caused a loss of hair, dab the affected area with diluted *Molkosan* and, after drying, dust with *Urticalcin* powder. This treatment usually helps to get rid of the infection in a short time.

Excessively oily hair is often a problem for young people during puberty. In the case of girls, this is generally due to a temporary disruption of the ovarian function. In order to help, the root cause must be treated. Warm underwear is recommended and warm herbal sitz-baths are necessary, to be taken every night until relief is achieved. If a woman's hair is too greasy, her hormone production is poor. In this case, it is important to treat the hormone glands, perhaps by taking a good homoeopathic preparation such as *Ovarium* and having regular sitz-baths in order to ensure good circulation. If the stagnation is serious, *Aesculus* will help rectify the trouble. Proceeding in this way will have an indirect beneficial influence on the hair. Moreover, if you follow this treatment, you will not only benefit your hair but also the general condition of your health, since many other body functions depend on the proper functioning of the glands.

It is remarkable what results one can achieve with hair problems. When I was about seven years old, during the Second World War, I was shot in the head. Fortunately I survived, but the bullet was millimetres from my brain and I was left with a hole in my head and a bald patch. The same German enemy who shot me tried to make up for it. Years later, I went to an exhibition in Germany and discovered a company called Stabil, who made shampoos and hair tonics. The practitioner on the stand pondered over my situation, but told me that I would never get my hair back. Nevertheless, he gave me a few things to try. To my great surprise, the hair returned to where I had had this bald patch for many years.

A great number of people consult me and write to me about their hair problems. I have been able to help loads of people by using the remedies I have already mentioned coupled with good guidance, and they enjoy healthy hair growth today.

Sometimes problems are caused by the blood circulation being impeded. If this is the problem, Indian head massage or head reflexology can be extremely beneficial, as can some pressure on the choroid plexus, which releases the cerebrospinal fluid.

Dr Rees of Sedan, Kansas, pioneered this treatment. Through temporal-sphenoid release (via carefully targeted cranial massage), he diverted the cerebrospinal fluid to the portion of the anatomy which had been deprived of its normal quota. The temporal-sphenoid ring is a master control panel for all nerve functions in the body, a type of logistic centre of supply and demand. It could even be the control centre that the psychologist uses via the subconscious mind to change body functions. All vascular and lymphatic reflexes will show up on the temporal-sphenoid line. Dr R.M. MacLain of Oakland, California, said a great many years ago: 'Any disturbance that may affect the choroid plexus would naturally affect either the quality or the quantity of the fluid that it secretes, and any fluctuation in this fluid would certainly influence its pressure. The normal pressure appears to have a stabilising effect upon the entire body.'

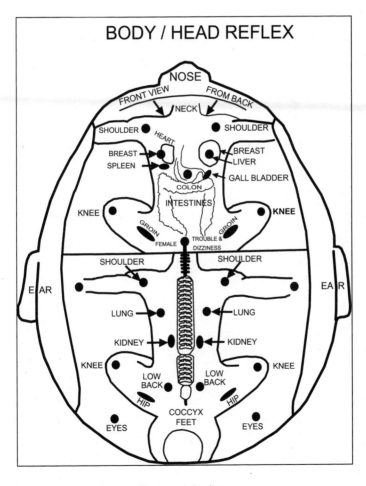

The cranial reflexes

So, we have now looked at the skin, hair and nails. Beauty from within is important. With the dietary management I have written about in this book, together with the introduction of remedies, it is amazing how much can be done to help alleviate problems in these areas.

CHAPTER FIVE

Allergies

In the days when I first studied medicine, a few books covered the subject of allergies; today, they could fill a library. People can become allergic to virtually anything in this day and age, however innocuous it might appear. Just the other day, I even spoke to a lady who told me she was allergic to her husband!

The word 'allergy' was first used in 1906, so why has this problem only become so overwhelming in the past few decades? Not so long ago, an allergy was something out of the ordinary; today, they are widespread. It is officially accepted that the contamination of our modern environment has created a climate conducive to the development of such illnesses. In our time, allergies, mainly to food, are increasing uncontrollably. Over 70 per cent of the population of the industrial countries have an allergic disposition.

Allergies can often be underestimated and we have found that not only can an allergy lead to multiple sclerosis or Alzheimer's disease but it can also cause other severe problems. We have possibly been a bit dismissive about the extent and seriousness of allergies in the past. I am at fault as well, because I previously thought of some minor allergies as not being very significant, but have since become more knowledgeable about the physical and mental disturbances allergies can cause. It is therefore vital that any problems are investigated. With the use of the Vegacheck machine, a quick analysis can be made of the patient's health from head to toe. This non-invasive device can detect disturbances or disorders within the body which are often not detectable by the use of other methods such as ultrasound, X-rays, CAT scans or laboratory blood tests. Machines like the Vegacheck, the Health Check, the Dermatron or the Vincent can pinpoint areas in need of attention and lead us to a problem that could possibly have been avoided. Prevention is always better than cure. In the next chapter, on the immune system, I shall explain why many allergies are triggered when the immune system becomes weak. In treating people with allergies, I always make a point of initially concentrating on the immune system. That is often all that is required to eliminate some allergies.

So what is an allergy? As I have said, I have written extensively on this subject in my book *Viruses, Allergies and the Immune System*. When speaking of an allergy, we mean 'a changed or unusual defensive reaction against a specific known or unknown substance'. An allergy is basically a hypersensitivity of the body to certain substances, proteins or foodstuffs that it is unable to accept or with which it is not compatible. An allergic disposition can be hereditary or acquired. An allergic reaction to a substance or to food can occur within seconds or over a period of up to 72 hours. Most affected are the skin and the mucus membranes. There is no need to describe here the very complicated process which can trigger an allergic reaction – this subject has often been described elsewhere. What we want to know is *why* we become allergic. Usually people become allergic because, for some reason, their liver is unable to detoxify the offending substances. This is often due to an overload of toxins.

Headaches, dizziness or migraine headaches that occur more or less regularly can be the first signs of an allergy. People who are suffering from bronchitis, sinusitis or asthma often owe their disease to an allergic disposition. The same applies in the case of tachycardia (a rapid heartbeat), shortage of breath and similar problems. Some other common problems are sore throats, ear infections, lymph-node swelling, digestive disorders, skin eruptions (especially eczema and hives), respiratory problems (from a runny nose to pneumonia), muscle and joint pains and abdominal pain. Usually there are mental disturbances at the same time. The earliest of these to manifest themselves when a person is suffering from an allergy are irritability, moodiness and sleep disorders, especially nightmares and night terrors. Some children become hyperactive and difficult to manage. Other children wilt and withdraw, developing symptoms similar to those displayed by autistic children.

Allergic reactions can occur as a result of milk and other dairy products, refined cane sugar, industrial cocoa, chocolate, corn, eggs, wheat, soy, citrus fruits (usually when they have been sprayed or waxed), monosodium glutamate, preservatives, dyes, caffeine, sweeteners, saturated fats, pork, sausages, eggs, breakfast cereals, tinned foods, strong cheese, margarine, cornflakes, peanuts, Brazil nuts, nicotine, Brussels sprouts, artichokes, Savoy cabbage, peas and hundreds of other things, including vegetables from the nightshade family, like tomatoes, aubergines and potatoes.

An allergic reaction can also be caused by an addiction to certain kinds of food. If, for example, a person loves to eat chocolate and eats this almost every day, certain defensive reactions against the very concentrated contents become overstrained. This reaction can be against the refined sugar, industrial cocoa or saturated fats contained within chocolate, and it becomes impossible for the organism to replace the specific defensive cells needed quickly enough. In this case, the body has to take other measures and any part of the body will cooperate in order to defend against the allergens – that is, substances with which our body can no longer cope. This situation can be compared to an army: when some special troops are unable to continue to fight, other units have to take over. The next battle will then perhaps be fought somewhere else, with different weapons. In our body, first there may be a reaction that affects the skin. Later reactions may take place deeper in the body. People who get allergic reactions after eating their favourite food should refrain from having it in the future.

Far more diseases are caused by allergens than we generally believe, so it is quite sad to see that the allergic response is often taken out of context. We have to realise that when a person becomes allergic, the immune system is often depressed, and that there are many causes that can trigger allergic reactions. Some simple allergy tests will reveal the cause, and it is often interesting to see how allergies disappear when the suspect foods are avoided or eliminated. Unfortunately, most doctors do not understand this and they treat, for example, any asthmatic reaction or bronchitis with medication which suppresses the symptoms. That the patient in question could be allergic to, say, cow's milk, sugar, chocolate, beer or certain chemical substances in the food is completely ignored. Because of this, millions of patients have to take suppressive medication their whole life. Any patient with chronic health problems should at least try to cut out of their diet, for one or two weeks, any food which they eat regularly. It is very possible that a health problem they have had for years will disappear completely when the offending substance is taken away.

Often it is not the food itself but the additives in the food which cause allergies. This explains why people are not always consistently allergic to the same food. If there are no additives in the food, there will be no allergic reactions. Not only can there be allergic reactions to ordinary food, but also to substances we come into contact with every day, such as cleaning fluids, aerosols or petrol fumes.

Allergies can develop at any time in life, even in babies. The digestive system of the baby was designed to deal with its mother's milk, which has a completely different quality and composition from cow's milk. The digestion of the foreign protein in cow's milk is far from easy for a baby, and the great surplus of phosphorus and other factors is also problematic. Often the organism excretes the offending substances through the skin and therefore many babies get skin problems, for example so-called milk crust. If these skin problems are not treated correctly, or the symptoms are suppressed by medication, very often more serious diseases may develop and the baby will retain an allergic disposition throughout its entire life. Such a baby will develop a great sensitivity to all kinds of things, not only to milk and milk products. Allergic reactions in infancy are expressed as crying, colic, excessive vomiting, diarrhoea, rashes, eczema and cold-like respiratory congestion.

During the years I have been in practice, I have often seen people who were extremely healthy but who suddenly became allergic to pollen and developed hay fever. If this troublesome allergy is left untreated, then the problem will get worse. However, one can do so much to bring relief to sufferers, even by the use of a simple remedy like *Luffa Complex* or *ALR-Formula* from Michael's. These remedies can help to get hay fever quickly under control, as well as rhinitis, sinusitis, conjunctivitis, asthma or any other bacterial problems. Self-help is at hand and one thing that is essential is to carry out detoxification and help improve one's immunity.

There are between 700 and 800 allergic substances for which skin-testing preparations, desensitising treatment and vaccines are available. Desensitising the system can be extremely effective. In straightforward cases, all that may be needed are homoeopathic remedies, such as

Luffa Complex or *Devil's Claw Extract* which can give brilliant results. By using more sophisticated methods, we can find out what is causing an allergy and then treat the underlying problem.

Do allergies really account for many of today's problems? I am convinced that they actually cause a lot more problems than we ever thought. Allergic reactions can be traced by watching for changes in behaviour patterns. Quite a while ago, I carried out some research work in men's and women's prisons in Britain which really opened my eyes to the enormity of the problems caused by allergies. The particular study I was carrying out in these prisons was to see if a link could be proven to exist between the diet of the prisoners and their behaviour, and I was staggered by the extent of their allergies. Surprisingly, I became quite fond of one particular fellow I treated, who had committed several murders. The extent of his allergies was shocking. After carrying out sensitivity tests using the Vegacheck machine, I asked him what he had eaten before committing his last horrific murder, which led to his imprisonment. He told me he had drunk several mugs of coffee, each containing six spoonfuls of sugar and lots of milk. He had not consumed much alcohol, but had eaten half a loaf of bread, smothered in jam. The Vegacheck machine can give an indication of what is going wrong in the system, and, interestingly, it revealed that he was extremely allergic to milk, coffee, sugar, chocolate, wheat and alcohol – almost all of which he had consumed before committing this appalling deed. It was enough to make him hyperactive and put him in a state of mind in which he was ready to commit murder.

As he continued consuming these offending products after being imprisoned, his behaviour, needless to say, showed no signs of improvement. Even the guards who brought him his food were afraid that he would have another outburst. Once the foodstuffs to which he was allergic were removed from his diet and I carried out some further work on him, he became a totally different person. He had improved so much that when Princess Anne visited the prison some time later, the prison officers told her about the transformation and she enquired as to what had changed him. He explained what had happened and said that all he wanted to do now was to make up for the dreadful life he had led and the awful deeds he had carried out. I saw him not so long ago, very happy and a valuable member of the community.

I have actually spoken about my research work in the House of Lords, and even pleaded for MPs to do something about the dietary management of prisoners. Many prisoners I had studied became so aggressive that they committed murder purely as a result of being on a totally wrong diet. I also spoke to female prisoners who, due to an imbalance in their hormone systems, had murdered the people they probably loved the most – their own husbands. In my book *Viruses, Allergies and the Immune System,* I dedicate a chapter to diet and mental health.

It is not until some people become concerned about a change in their mental state that they consult me, and it is often only then that the discovery is made that they have severe allergies. Fortunately, at my clinic, with the use of our Vegacheck machine and the Health Check machine, which gives a general overview of patients' health, we can get a clear indication of where allergy and health problems lie. It takes a lot of time and effort to go through the allergy testing process, but a successful outcome makes it all worthwhile.

THE ALLERGY RIDDLE

The allergy problem is very complex. According to some physicians, hyperactivity and behavioural problems have nothing to do with allergic reactions. That, of course, is a matter of opinion. It is undeniable that there is usually not one cause but rather several (often overlapping) ones. Allergic reactions have been thought of differently through the ages, and the most recent explanations of them are so complicated that only a specialist physician could easily find their way through the maze.

A hundred years ago, hardly anybody would have thought that mental diseases, physical problems or unusual behaviour could have anything to do with a reaction to certain foods or substances in foods. This changed when some doctors in North America, Britain and, later, Germany started to look into these problems. Scientists like Theron Randolph, Herbert Rinkel, Albert Rowe, George Watson, Professor Comrey, Richard Mackarness, Professor Pfister, Lothar Burgerstein, Anna Calantin and many others achieved outstanding results by treating food allergies. Their accomplishments were so amazing that we should never overlook them. In his clinic near London, Richard Mackarness treated and cured countless allergic patients. It is not only modern doctors who have looked to nutrition for answers. We know that Hippocrates, as early as 460 BC, and other famous doctors of antiquity were convinced that mental diseases and abnormal behaviour were often caused by a malfunction of the metabolism and not by a sick mind or a bad or unbalanced personality. Even in those early times, patients improved when their eating habits were changed and they were treated with laxatives or emetics.

Knowing all this, we are able to draw some conclusions. Firstly, long ago some abnormal diseases were caused by the wrong metabolic reactions, and this means that some people, even in those times, could not digest certain foods. Of course, in 460 BC food additives and chemical pollution of the environment were non-existent, but it is exactly these that are mainly responsible for the vast increase in behavioural problems and mental diseases in our time.

In Hippocratic times, most food was still natural. However, people soon realised that oil- or fat-containing food did not taste good after a while, as it became rancid. Today, oil is still a difficult problem. Rancid oil is inedible and dangerous for our health. However, when oil has been exposed to high temperatures, it becomes saturated and loses its healthy qualities. Cold-pressed oil, extracted during the first pressing of olives or other oleaginous fruit and vegetables, can still become rancid if measures are not taken to prevent this. Bottles should be hermetically sealed and should be stored in a dark place, as light can spoil these very sensitive oils. All manufacturers of industrially heated oils fear rancidity, and therefore add several additives to oil, butter and other fatty and perishable food.

It is quite possible that, in olden times, people were not allergic to foods themselves but to the rancid fats in food. Milk, too, soon becomes spoiled when it has not been heated. In the past, many newborn babies died when their mothers were unable to feed them and they were given animal milk. This had much to do with the unhygienic conditions in which the milk was kept in those times.

Today, these problems have increased many times over, as most foods children like, even if they themselves can be metabolised, contain additives and other toxic substances. It is almost impossible to find food that is not contaminated. Even 'natural' fruit and vegetables often come from soil that is full of chemicals and lacks the most important nutrients. Most fruit and vegetables are sprayed and packed into plastic or other wrappings or containers made from artificial, toxic materials, which can leak into the food. Years ago, my great friend Maurice Hanssen wrote a book on E numbers and additives, giving invaluable guidance and advice to anyone who was searching for it. Following its publication, everyone realised the effect that E numbers had on the human body, and it sent shock waves through the food industry.

We should not forget that the body needs a lot of energy to fight against the flood of dangerous chemicals we face in modern life. This energy is badly needed for defence against disease and other important tasks. It is extremely important to find out what kind of foods or substances you are sensitive or allergic to so that you can omit them and at least try to prevent the loss of energy which consuming them incurs.

If you suspect, for instance, that your child might be allergic to a food he eats quite often, you should cut it out completely from his diet for four or five days, and then try a little of this food, no more than a teaspoonful, on the child's empty stomach in the morning. If there is a negative reaction, like a headache, a rapid heartbeat, vomiting or other signs of feeling unwell, you should no longer give your child that particular food. You can test many different kinds of food and in this way find out which of them causes a reaction.

Testing at home has its advantages and often the results of such tests can help you very much indeed. In some hospitals and clinics which specialise in food allergies or similar problems, the same kind of method is used. In my clinic, patients are often put on a so-called water fast for a few days. During this time, they are not allowed to eat anything – they drink only water, so that their digestive tract becomes as clean as possible. After that, the testing begins.

FOOD ALLERGIES AND INTOLERANCES

Food allergies are quite easy to detect, but it is far more difficult to detect intolerance to a certain food. The symptoms can become evident up to 30 hours or more after the questioned ingredient has been introduced. In the case of hyperactivity or difficulty in prolonged concentration, food intolerance should be a suspect. Experts say that at least one in every two children suffers from intolerance to one or more food substances.

The blood test for allergies does not reveal this problem. One indication may be an extreme addiction to a particular food or drink. Children may become irritable or impatient if they cannot have it.

The same thing happens when a drug addict stops taking drugs – this is a symptom of withdrawal crisis! Children with food intolerances tend to become picky eaters with strong food preferences, refusing to eat many healthy foods. They typically become eating specialists, compulsively eating a small number of favourite foods. Vegetables are often the first foods rejected.

A patient I saw the other day had a nasty case of blepharitis, or inflammation of the eyelids. After carrying out some tests, I discovered that it was due to a reaction to cow's milk. When this was eliminated from the diet, the condition cleared up quickly. We often see that dermatitis, eczema, urticaria, photosensitivity or even colds can be cured by removing cow's milk from the diet.

While I was writing this chapter, a lady came to see me at my clinic. The poor soul was suffering from urticaria, an itchy rash – the worst case I have ever seen. Even in the middle of the night, she would go outside into the freezing cold in an attempt to alleviate the itching, which had become insufferable. When I carried out a test, I found that she was allergic to fresh, raw vegetables and fruit. When the Vegacheck machine detected what the allergy was, I immediately asked her to cut out all fresh vegetables and fresh fruit from her diet but to steam them instead, and also to eat dried fruit instead of fresh fruit. This went totally against my principles, as I always advocate the eating of fresh fruit and vegetables. However, as soon as she did this, the condition cleared up.

The other day, I saw a patient who had a nasty case of laryngitis. After carrying out the necessary tests, it was discovered that she had severe allergic reactions to fungi. Once again, by omitting the suspect food from her diet – in this case mushrooms – the problem disappeared.

It is so rewarding when I see the successes I have had with patients who have sometimes gone to great lengths to get to the bottom of their allergies. Their problems have totally cleared up by simply removing the offending substance from their lives – whether it be a foodstuff, everyday dust or house mites, or something more unusual.

In the medical profession, we need to take problems like allergies and intolerances more seriously. It seems to be all the rage to say, 'I have an intolerance to such and such', using it as an excuse for something or other. Nevertheless, patients should always be taken seriously in order to find out exactly what the problem is.

ALLERGENS

As a result of modern agricultural and cattle-breeding methods, it is not only industrial products which contain allergens – natural ones can, too. One can have an allergic reaction to almost anything and such a reaction can take place in any part of the body. An allergic disposition can lie dormant for many years and break out only after the person in question comes into contact with certain allergens while their defensive forces are under par.

Phosphates in Food

At the beginning of the twentieth century, there were only a few food additives on the market; nowadays there are thousands of them, as well as innumerable foreign substances from the environment. It is logical that the human organism tries to defend itself against all these toxins. Even when a certain substance is harmless in itself, it is possible that through its combination with other additives new and often very toxic substances can come into being. In medicine, these dangers are known and many books have been written on the subject, but in the food industry, they are completely ignored.

Some of the food additives used most frequently today are phosphates, which are considered harmless by the official authorities provided that the daily intake is no more than 750 mg. Phosphates really can work miracles. Using these chemicals, dull, unattractive, old and wilted food can be made to look fresh and appetising. Phosphates are used in the cheese and meat industries, and in manufacturing cakes, pastries, soups, sauces, chocolate, soft drinks and so on. They have excellent qualities as buffers, emulsifiers, thickening agents, coagulators and water absorbents, and are also used to render certain substances inactive.

The foods which children like best are embellished and improved by phosphates in order to make them more attractive. Sausages, hamburgers, soft drinks, ice cream, pastries, sweets, puddings – everything contains phosphates. Therefore children often consume more than twice the amount recommended for adults.

Symptoms from an overdose of phosphates are often quite serious. One of these is MCD, minimal cerebral dysfunction. Other symptoms are hyperactivity, hypoactivity and autism. Hyperactive children fidget all the time and never keep quiet. Hypoactive and autistic children, on the contrary, lose all *joie de vivre* and seem to have no energy at all. Children who suffer from an allergy to phosphates will usually display some of the following symptoms:

- Antisocial behaviour
- Disturbed muscular functions and uncontrolled movements
- Congenital alexia: spelling and reading problems
- Lack of concentration, inability to listen
- Fear of physical contact
- Osteoporosis, disorders of bone-healing
- Pylorus cramps: cramps of the stomach muscles
- Pseudo croup: coughing fits because of restricted air passage
- Disorders of the heart muscle
- Allergies: asthma, hay fever, nettle rash, eczema
- Various skin diseases, e.g. neurodermatitis

- Vasomotoric disorders, e.g. migraine
- Disorders of the stomach and intestinal dysfunctions
- Ulcers of the stomach or ulcers of the duodenum

Hertha Hafer, the author of the book *The Hidden Drug: Dietary Phosphate,* gives the reader many sound arguments and proofs of the dangers of phosphates. There has been much scientific research on this subject but, for several reasons, most of this has not been published or has simply been ignored. Certainly, not all of the symptoms mentioned above result only from an overdose of phosphates, and every disease has more than one cause, but it is high time the situation was researched more thoroughly. Not only children but also adults become ill and suffer because of the irresponsible attitude of food manufacturers.

Metals

When children suffer from problems such as ADD (attention deficit disorder), AD/HD (attention deficit/hyperactivity disorder), hyperactivity, autism, learning disabilities, irritability and other mental problems, as well as allergies, tummy-aches and constipation, the cause is an accumulation of heavy and toxic metals in combination with other negative factors and influences. By and large, lead, mercury, aluminium, copper and cadmium are the most dangerous toxic metals, and all day long we are in contact with these metals without realising the danger.

Lead

Lead is still being used in many industrial plants. We absorb lead by drinking contaminated water or by breathing polluted air. Many old houses still have lead pipes. There may be lead in your toothpaste tube, and that lead will be assimilated by the toothpaste and get into your body. Newspaper ink contains lead, and it is also to be found in insecticides, fungicides, some commercial baby milk, many different kinds of fish, offal, cosmetics, hair colourings, paper clips, cooking utensils, glassware, some paints, wine, cigarette smoke and in parks where children play. When you smoke a cigarette, you can relax while getting some nice lead arsenate (used on tobacco crops as an insecticide) into your lungs. Although the use of lead in petrol is no longer permitted, exhaust fumes from cars can still endanger our health in other ways.

Some of the symptoms of lead poisoning are impotence, sterility, birth defects, insomnia, anaemia, muscle weakness, constipation or diarrhoea, headaches, depression, fatigue and irritability. When even small quantities of lead accumulate in the body, a child may suffer from fatigue, growth problems, restlessness, muscle weakness, mental retardation, learning difficulties, loss of appetite, anorexia, confusion, impaired motor-skill development, behavioural disorders, irritability and behaviour changes.

Mercury

Thimerosal, the mercury-containing compound used in amalgam fillings, can leak out from these. Mercury fillings become highly potent neurotoxins, easily absorbed by nerve cells. These toxins infiltrate the brain, as well as other parts of the body, within 24 hours. We may also find mercury in laxatives, cosmetics and prescription drugs. There is often mercury in fabric softeners. Mercury is even in some hepatitis B and DPT vaccines! Many large kinds of fish, like tuna or salmon, fresh or tinned, may contain mercury. Chemical fertilisers, pesticides, fungicides, water-based paints and even fluorescent lights are often made with mercury.

As a consequence of the accumulation of this metal, there is emotional instability, depression, fatigue, poor concentration, memory loss and hypertension. Mercury can cause kidney damage, tremors, loss of hearing and vision, sore gums, gingivitis and headaches. Even small quantities can provoke mental retardation, skin eruptions, chronic fatigue, learning disabilities, apathy, drowsiness, nervousness, chromosome damage and AD/HD in children. There is an interesting degree of similarity between the symptoms of mercury poisoning and those of autism.

Removing amalgam fillings from your teeth can be dangerous if your dentist does not know how to go about it properly. A dentist who is really health conscious will be sure to do it very carefully so that as little mercury as possible enters into the bloodstream, from where it could get into the rest of the body.

Aluminium

Aluminium can be found in many deodorants, in cookware and in construction materials. Kettles can be made from aluminium, copper or other metals, and even the table salt we use for our egg in the morning contains some aluminium in order to keep the salt dry. The metal is still used in aerosol sprays and kitchen foil. There is even aluminium in our food (in emulsifiers), in beer and soft-drink cans and in pharmaceutical drugs, such as antacids and many others. The aluminium silicates from aerosol sprays can be directly transported through nerve connections from the nose into the brain and deposited in the most sensitive areas. According to a report in *The Lancet* in 1989, many infant formulas contain aluminium. Human breast milk may contain 5–20 micrograms of aluminium per litre, but there is 20 times as much in some formulas based on cow's milk, and there can be 100 times as much in soy-based formulas. Breast milk is still the safest milk by far.

Aluminium can cause headaches, brain degeneration, senile dementia and gastritis. In small children, it may be the cause of gas, colic, motor and behavioural dysfunction, skin rashes and nervousness. Aluminium is known to inhibit and reduce an important co-factor in the synthesis of many neurotransmitters. It also promotes acute psychotic conditions by making the blood–brain barrier more permeable to ingested neurotoxins.

My third daughter is highly trained in allergy testing of the whole body. Using the Vegacheck machine, she discovered that patients showing signs of Alzheimer's disease were allergic to quite a number of substances and, most interestingly, some exhibited a strong allergic reaction to aluminium. Extensive testing has been carried out in America on Alzheimer's disease in relation to cooking with aluminium pans. For years, when I have taken blood tests of Alzheimer patients, I too have detected the presence of aluminium. Sadly, that particular research has not been further developed. I believe, however, that this problem is getting worse. As much as we hear about the increase in cancer, the same is also happening with Alzheimer's disease. After I became aware of this research, when I was presented with patients who were showing the first signs of Alzheimer's disease or senility, I looked into their allergy situation thoroughly. I hear too often about the escalation of these diseases nowadays and I feel strongly that dietary management, blood circulation and many other factors should be carefully explored. I am aware that Alzheimer's might be inherited, but, nevertheless, it is essential to have it thoroughly checked in order to find out where the problem lies – could it be amalgam fillings, aluminium or copper levels, or even lead poisoning?

Copper

Copper levels in the blood rise when zinc levels drop, as happens in females the week before their period and when on contraceptive pills. Copper levels also rise in both sexes when sugar is eaten. Copper comes from birth-control pills, copper water pipes, water heaters, pesticides, brewery equipment, salt, alcoholic beverages, meats (it is used in animals as a growth enhancer) and soya beans, in which levels are very high.

While copper is an essential trace mineral needed by our body, exposure to too great a quantity of copper may overstimulate the brain and cause an insufficiency of zinc, hair loss, anaemia, arthritis, insomnia, poor concentration, irritability, hypertension, post-partum psychosis, toxaemia in pregnancy, inflammation of the liver, and, in children, digestive disorders, colic and behavioural problems. High copper levels can increase the chances of a child developing cystic fibrosis. In schizophrenics, copper levels are usually elevated.

When the excess of copper has been removed by chelation – treatment with a substance which combines with toxins to render them harmless – there is usually a rapid improvement. When copper is eliminated from the body, as a reaction to the cleansing efforts you may get acne. Acne will break out where the copper stores are being depleted, for example, around your mouth, neck or chest. When these surplus metals are gone from the body, the acne will disappear. Zinc helps to counteract some of the harmful effects of copper.

Cadmium

Cadmium is still found in some water pipes and in cigarettes, fertilisers, soft-drink dispensers, old dental fillings, refined foods and some metal containers, and it can leak from plastics. It can cause emphysema, kidney and liver damage, nephritis, abdominal cramps, colic, slow healing (because of a zinc deficiency), anaemia, acne and hypertension, and it is known to be a zinc antagonist. The cadmium in cigarette smoke is very dangerous. It is not only toxic for the smoker but also for the non-smoker, especially for children.

Vanadium

Vanadium is contained in relatively high levels in milk, egg whites, gelatine and shellfish. It is a heavy metal which, in trace amounts, seems to be essential for us. When vanadium is elevated in the blood and the hair, severe depression may occur. In this case, a supplement of ascorbic acid can be very helpful. Vanadium can prevent the transport of sodium across cell membranes. This means that the sodium content inside the cells becomes too high and cells cannot build up the full electric potential required for proper functioning. If blood pressure is low, apathy, memory impairment and social withdrawal can result.

In dealing with this large-scale problem of allergies, it is important that we do everything we possibly can to bring problems under control or, better still, eliminate them. It may perhaps only take some simple remedies to clear up an allergy, but if there is waste material in the human body that needs to be removed, then it is crucial that this is attended to. Strong remedies such as *Blood Detoxification Factors* by Michael's, *Doctor's Choice Antioxidant* by Enzymatic or Vogel's *Detox Box* might be necessary to improve matters. It is imperative to find out where an allergy lies. If left untreated, a small allergy problem could lead to a serious degenerative disease. Conditions such as rheumatism, arthritis, multiple sclerosis, muscular dystrophy or Alzheimer's disease can all result from allergic reactions.

Because the incidence of Alzheimer's disease is rapidly increasing, I want to devote some of this book to this massive subject.

ALZHEIMER'S DISEASE

Although more and more people suffer from Alzheimer's disease and, because of this, much scientific research has been done, nobody, as yet, has found any definite indication as to the cause of this illness. Deficient genetic material most probably has something to do with the development of Alzheimer's. However, it may take decades until science will be more advanced in this respect and the right therapy becomes available. In the meantime, in Europe, as well as in the United States, the majority of patients are treated only for their symptoms;

most of the remedies used hardly do any good and indeed they can even harm the patient.

Not only during treatment but also during diagnosis, the doctors concerned are interested chiefly in the brain. It is there that the so-called 'plaques' – protein-containing diseased areas which are a characteristic feature of Alzheimer's – can be found, as well as nerve fibres which seem to be 'glued' together. Many scientific and popular papers and books have been written about all this, so there is no need here for more explanation.

As there is no known cause, medicine can only treat these patients by way of physiotherapy, occupational therapy and medication. Psychotherapy might be useful in the early stages of the disease.

Mens Sana in Corpore Sano

This does not only mean 'a healthy mind in a healthy body'; it also means that body and mind are one and cannot be separated. When a person is no longer able to think logically, when they are totally mixed up and do not even recognise their closest relatives, then not only the brain but the entire organism is ill. Our brain, like other parts of the body and the organs, gets its nourishment from the blood. When the blood does not contain all the special nutrients the brain needs, brain cells cannot develop normally any more. When the blood contains an ever-increasing quantity of toxins and therefore less oxygen reaches the brain, many brain cells will weaken or die.

It seems logical that the brain is more sensitive than other parts of the body and reacts in a more powerful way when there is a lack of nutrients or when there are too many toxins. Although blood levels may be completely normal, nevertheless there may be some interneuronal or intercellular lack of certain specific substances.

Because of our modern eating habits, we are in great danger. The mass production of food is primarily aimed at benefiting the industry.

The cheapest way in which to guarantee a long shelf-life is to sacrifice nutrients. Because of this, especially in the USA, scientific research increased in the last century in respect of the link between poor nutrition and mental diseases and diseases of the elderly. This research laid the foundations for orthomolecular medicine – preventing and treating illness through optimum nutrition – which has now become an official medical discipline and can be identified as strictly scientific.

Orthomolecular psychiatry in the USA and in the UK is very successful. Years ago, Dr Carl C. Pfeiffer of the well-known Brain Bio Center in New Jersey could show a healing quotient of 85–100 per cent with his schizophrenic patients. In treating not only schizophrenia but also other mental diseases, very high doses of vitamins, minerals, trace elements, essential amino and fatty acids and other vital substances are given to the patients. In order to find out individual deficiencies, patients are checked first for food allergies, for lack of special nutrients and for heavy metals, amongst other things. The patient is tested for about 50 different substances. When there is a lack of certain B vitamins, the person in question may have become confused, irritable, depressive or sleepless, and may suffer from a loss of memory.

Because of earlier treatment with antibiotics, the intestinal flora of the patients can be so badly damaged that, as a result, there is fungal disease. When important intestinal bacteria disappear, fungi (candida) can multiply freely. As fungi cannot help with the digestion of our food, this, in turn, causes a lack of nutrients, so that the candida toxins add an additional strain. According to Dr W.G. Crook in *Yeasts and How They Can Make You Sick,* this can even cause autism in children. There is more and more proof for the theory that the general health of the patient and the condition of their intestinal flora are closely related to diseases of the brain and to many other health problems. All brain diseases are, at least partly, caused by a faulty metabolism.

Dr Theron Randolph from Chicago described how when eating

habits are changed, psychological disorders sometimes clear up completely. Professor Dieter Häussinger from Freiburg has written that the 'toxin hypothesis' is making progress in scientific circles and is becoming widely accepted. This hypothesis says that ammonia and other substances from the intestines can bypass the liver. These will be insufficiently detoxified and then enter the blood-circulation system, and hence the brain. This superfluous ammonia, which cannot be rendered harmless, has neurotoxic properties.

Ammonia is only one example. All poisons which cannot be broken down or eliminated enter into the blood and become harmful to our health. On the other hand, as a result of modern denaturalised nutrition, our bodies suffer from an ever-growing lack of vital substances.

Dr Konrad Beyreuther, Dean of Biological Molecular Medicine at Heidelberg University, Germany, asserts that 'a long life, semi-luxury food and stimulants', which are at variance with the science of nutrition, are the cause of the rapidly increasing progress of Alzheimer's disease. Such patients are probably undersupplied with vitamins E and C and beta-carotene, as well as trace elements such as selenium, manganese, copper and zinc (the so-called 'radical traps'). In his opinion, free radicals (which can develop when there is a lack of certain vital nutrients) cause the development in the brain of those amyloid plaques typical of Alzheimer's, which destroy communication between the nerve cells. In order to prevent this development, he recommends the intake of the above-mentioned vitamins and other vital substances. In principle, all nutrition should be as natural as possible and contain sufficient raw vegetables and fruits, as well as different natural oils, seeds and nuts.

Summary

In order to prevent Alzheimer's disease and when treating patients suffering from it, it is to be recommended that:

- patients should not receive any further toxic substances or be exposed to them
- all nutrition should be as natural and untreated as possible
- nutrients in which patients are deficient should be supplied

It has been shown above that the composition of the blood has much to do with so-called mental diseases and therefore also with Alzheimer's disease. As a result, more and more physicians recommend wholesome nutrition and multivitamin therapy, whereby sometimes a worsening of the disease may be prevented.

However, such a disease does not develop in the space of a few days. By and by, the composition of the blood changes. When there is a steady influx of substances which, as Dr Konrad Beyreuther says, 'are at variance with the science of nutrition', the digestive system will be more and more overburdened so that some toxins will get into the bloodstream. As Professor Lothar Wendt has shown, the blood will be more and more saturated by toxins and tiny particles will stick to the walls of the blood vessels. In the long run, these deposits will increase in size. Some of these substances will even permeate the blood–brain barrier, the protective network of blood vessels and cells that filters blood flowing to the brain. Toxins will then get into the fine capillaries of the brain, where they will be responsible for much damage.

Of course, a personal predisposition (genetic or acquired), a weak defence mechanism, former diseases, injuries, health problems such as alcoholism, smoking, industrial toxins, head injuries and too much stress also play a role here. A further consequence of this blood condition, which in the vernacular is called 'thick blood', is that the blood cannot transport sufficient oxygen to the brain. And everyone knows that our brain needs a great deal of oxygen!

Although it is very important to try, through optimal nutrition, healthy living and the avoidance wherever possible of toxins, to hold up the development of the disease, it would be even more wonderful to be able to prevent it or to reverse the disease in its early stages. However, according to modern medicine, Alzheimer's disease is incurable. In olden times, on the other hand, mental diseases were not classified straightaway as being 'incurable'. This only happened when the patient was extremely old or when their defences were so low that treatment would have been useless.

The brain was always considered as part of the entire human being, of the entire organism. In the case of mental disturbances, many different cleansing methods, by way of perspiration and stimulation of the skin, by enemas or purges and laxatives, as well as bleeding and so on, were already known to the Egyptians. Many years ago, reflexology, as in modern times, was already known in India. In those days, the arsenal of available therapies was much larger and, in the case of each disease, the whole body was treated, not only the diseased organ or part, as is so often the case nowadays. In olden times, every physician knew about natural connections and therefore many diseases which today are classified as incurable were treated successfully.

All this knowledge was taught in the medical schools of Knidos and of Kos, from where Hippocrates, the 'father of medicine', came. He taught us that natural healing forces encouraged by increased elimination, such as vomiting, defecation, sputum, perspiration, bleeding from the nose, from haemorrhoids or through menstruation, pus and skin rashes can, in a functional and purposeful way, overcome disease. Hippocrates thought of the physician as a servant of nature, who should follow the ways indicated by nature to heal. Many great and famous physicians of olden and modern times, like

Hippocrates, Galen, Maimonides, Paracelsus, Hufeland, Kneipp, Aschner, Boerhaave, Brauchle, Bircher-Benner and many others, were convinced that the treatment of disease without elimination of surplus or diseased fluids – which today we call toxic substances – would not be possible. 'Healing is cleaning' was the conclusion arrived at through observations and experience at the sickbed.

In recent times, the healing of many diseases, especially chronic and mental ones, has become very problematic or even impossible, because the fundamental and deeper-lying causes can no longer be recognised and therefore cannot be used therapeutically.

By using those cleaning methods and in treating the entire organism, physicians in olden times were, without any doubt, more successful in treating mental diseases than they are nowadays. The belief in localised pathology during the last century has brought about a loss of understanding of natural connections between all bodily processes.

Bernard Aschner, one of the most famous physicians at the beginning of the last century, wrote:

> One should never believe that the physicians from the past centuries could not diagnose and heal mental diseases, and it is very depressing that most mental diseases could – in their early stages – be cured quickly and with ease by the right physical treatment.

All the time, there is proof of the fact that we are on the wrong track. In the case of Alzheimer's disease, nobody would ever think of cleansing the organism or treating the person's entire body. Nobody even gives this a thought and many physicians simply do not believe in such things. This is because modern textbooks do not mention anything about this. However, especially these days when we have so many new possibilities, we could achieve a great deal in this way.

Formerly, physicians observed that in the case of mental problems the digestive system does not usually function well. The patient might suffer from constipation, gastric weakness or other problems, or liver problems, or the intestinal flora might have been destroyed. They also observed an absence of menstruation in women suffering from mental problems. On the other hand, it was seen that in the case of bloody diarrhoea or loss of blood through some other cause, some mentally ill patients were cured. Only recently, scientific research has shown how extremely important the quality of the blood is in many kinds of disease.

Although many people realise how important healthy nutrition and, in some cases, certain nutrients are, this is only part of the picture. By giving the patient the right food and nutrients, the development of the disease may be somewhat held up. However, as long as nothing has been done concerning the elimination of toxins, no treatment can ever be really successful. As already mentioned, a disease like Alzheimer's does not develop overnight. Usually it takes decades until, through an excess of negative influences, the defensive forces of the body grow weaker and the disease can develop. Such a thing would never happen if the person concerned were really healthy and the composition of their blood in order. Only when health is already deteriorating and the blood becomes thick-flowing and full of toxins does the situation become dangerous.

How can one succeed in helping such a patient – even when their eating habits have been changed for the better – when their blood is still thick, the blood vessels are full of toxic deposits, when all over the body there are sediments in the connective tissues, when the skin cannot breathe any more and the patient cannot really perspire, when the stools and digestion are not in order, when the organs are so weak that they cannot fulfil their tasks, when the cells do not receive the right nourishment and when the entire organism is weak and full of toxins? In this case, the brain, day by day, will still be attacked by toxic material and the disease will worsen, so that therapy can only be a case of 'patching up'.

Unfortunately, medicine has forgotten the art of healing. True healing is time-consuming and can cost a lot of money, and therefore it is no longer taught at universities. However, the suppression of symptoms has nothing to do with healing and, on the contrary, always entails more illness. We have forgotten the guiding principle of the ancient physicians: 'to heal is to clean'. Although the Hippocratic oath is still very highly thought of, the healing methods of Hippocratic times, which for thousands of years have been repeatedly proven to work, are no longer or only seldom used, and most doctors do not know anything about them. This is a great pity, as many medical problems of our day could be solved by these methods of healing.

Only when the sick body has been carefully cleansed on all levels does the blood become lighter and flow with ease. Only then can one start thinking about the reconstruction of health. In the first place, the digestive system should be treated. The stools should be regulated and it should be made possible for the intestinal flora to recover. In order to allow this, the liver should be supported by natural medication. The lymphatic system should be treated and the natural defensive forces of the body should be made to function again. Also, the skin should be stimulated. Accordingly, the physician should fall back on the medical literature of the beginning of the last century as, particularly in the 10 to 30 years before the triumphant arrival of antibiotics and symptomatic medicine, medical science had made enormous progress, which was then suddenly swept under the carpet.

Now that many of us have realised that a repeated suppression of symptoms does not get us any further, we should look again for new (or old) ways to help patients without doing them any harm. As we do this, we will certainly find evidence that the ancient physicians were right after all when they said 'to heal is to clean'.

Practical Advice Regarding Alzheimer Patients
Diagnosis

Apart from the usual diagnosis, it is very important with Alzheimer patients to also check for food allergies and other allergic reactions. Furthermore, it is important to look for harmful substances, such as heavy metals, and to look for a lack of vitamins, minerals and other vital substances. Analysing the hair, blood and urine is therefore important. The hair analysis should be done first.

Further important questions

- What are the eating and drinking habits of the patient?
- Does the patient suffer from headaches or migraines?
- Does the patient have circulation problems (e.g. cold hands or feet)?
- How, and for how long, does the patient sleep?
- Does the patient perspire freely?
- Are there any problems urinating?
- Does the patient have regular bowel movements? What about the colour and consistency of the stools?
- Does the patient take enough outdoor exercise?

Without any doubt, the inner life of the patient is also extremely important. Vital questions would be, for example:

- How is the patient's family life?
- Did the patient have a goal in life?
- What kind of work did the patient do?

In the early stages of the disease, group therapy could be helpful. Frequent conversation with the patient is useful. The patient should never be bored, and occupational therapy is important as long as the patient is able to participate. In the event that the patient suffers from headaches or migraines, it is recommended, in the course of three weeks, to make notes concerning all eating and drinking habits. Often problems such as depression or nervous behaviour can be caused totally or partly by certain foods.

Therapeutic recommendations

The cleansing of the organism is most important. The objective of this kind of therapy is the purification of the organism on all levels. It does not make sense, for example, to clean the blood while the intestines are still full of toxins. Also, it is not very logical to clean only the intestines when the walls of the blood vessels remain full of deposits and the blood is dark and thick-flowing. In such a case, the brain cells are still supplied with toxic material. 'Healing' will always remain a form of art and only a physician who can understand the healing ways of nature itself will know when and how to use certain therapies and natural medication.

At home, as well as in a clinic, patients can be carefully introduced to cleansing treatments. Some of the changes to the living and eating habits of the patient should not be made too rapidly because when many toxins, some of which may have been in the body for decades, are being dissolved, it can happen that too many toxic substances will get into the blood at the same time and this can trigger unwanted and even dangerous reactions. This detoxification should be done slowly, step by step. Unfortunately, it is difficult to find a doctor who offers an intensive cleansing treatment, such as colon hydrotherapy, in their practice. However, more and more patients want such treatments and, as in any other profession, where there is a demand for something, the supply will increase.

In so far as the patient is still capable of understanding, they should personally be prepared for this cleansing process. They should try to understand how important this is, and relax and look forward to a possible improvement in their state of health. Positive thoughts are always helpful during treatment.

While the patient is still at home, relatives can do much to prevent the disease from worsening too rapidly and, as a result of this, care for the patient will be easier. Below are some recommendations for treatment during the first stages of Alzheimer's disease, which might prepare the patient for the ensuing, more intensive treatment. Of course, not all recommendations and methods of treatment can easily be followed, and it would be advantageous to choose those treatments which agree best with the patient.

It is important that the patient is in familiar surroundings. Simple, natural meals which do not burden the patient are also an important condition. Every human being is influenced by their everyday nutrition, on which their moods, behaviour, health or sickness partly depend, and which, in the case of any disease, is most important.

The following are some guidelines for treatment:

- While talking quietly to the patient, it is good to hold their hands and to caress them lightly.
- **Music therapy** This means listening to music which the patient enjoys, through headphones or speakers, the listening time depending on the patient. Music should never become tiring.
- **Colour therapy** Using certain colours to which the patient has a positive reaction. These colours should be included in the surroundings. This can either calm or stimulate the patient. There are also coloured glasses and other therapeutic possibilities.
- **Aromatherapy** Introducing specific scents which the patient likes. Certain scents have a direct influence on the mood and on the

human brain. Smelling is a very complicated and important process, the effects of which people have only lately started to understand.

- A light **brush massage** – always in the direction of the heart. This is very good for blood circulation. Some other types of massage are helpful too, but not classical massage, which is too drastic.

- A light **vibration massage** or **kinesiologic treatment** (such as putting the hands on the head, over the eyes and ears, and making light stroking movements) is very relaxing.

- **Massaging the tummy** can be very helpful, especially when there are problems of bowel movement.

- Some simple forms of **hydrotherapy**, such as a Kneipp herbal bath or foot baths (slowly increasing the temperature or alternating hot and cold baths), as well as arm baths. This is good for blood circulation and supports healing.

- At least twice a day, **the hair should be brushed lightly** for some time.

- **Sunbathing and light-bathing** or, when the weather is cold, a good sunlamp or other light therapy can be advantageous.

- **Humid compresses** on the tummy after eating, as in the Priessnitz regime, can help digestion.

- **Massaging the ears** is important for blood circulation to the brain.

- **Light gymnastics**

- Lying on a '**slant board**' (if the patient can do this without feeling dizzy), whereby the feet are about 30 cm higher than the head, will relieve the strain which is normally on many parts of the body. This should be practised at least three times a day, starting with five five-minute sessions and increasing the time to about twenty minutes.

- Light **massages with olive oil** or etheric oils can be carried out in order to loosen up toxic deposits in the back or, particularly, the stomach.

- **Homoeopathic remedies** or **phytotherapy** (treatment with plant-based medicines).

After one or two weeks, this treatment should be continued with the addition of:

- **Laxatives** or, when needed, other similar measures.
- **Schröpfen** (a therapeutic method whereby the skin is sucked into a glass in order to improve circulation – this is called 'cupping').
- **Oxygen therapy.**
- Special **foot baths** (with increasing heat).

Later, more therapies controlled by a physician who specialises in:

- **Colon hydrotherapy.**
- **HOT (hyperbaric oxygen treatment) detoxification**, while mixing the blood with oxygen.
- **Vapour baths**, perhaps a sauna.
- **Injections of the patient's own blood** (to encourage self-defence reactions).
- **Schlenz baths** (immersion of the body in a bathtub while the temperature of the water is steadily increased).
- **Perspiration treatments** (after taking laxatives or a Schlenz bath).
- **Bloodletting.**
- **Baunscheidt therapy** (scoring the skin slightly then rubbing in oil).

There are many other methods of treatment, including acupuncture, Bach flower remedies, neural therapy (very important to rebalance the energy flow), enzyme therapy and organ therapy.

An example of the daily programme

In the early stages of the disease, the daily programme for each patient and the different ways of treatment will always be based on personal needs and/or requirements. It would be ideal if two patients could more or less follow the same programme so that it would be a kind of challenge for both patients.

7 a.m.: Stretching and yawning in bed. The patient might massage their head and brush their hair in order to increase the blood circulation. They might also massage their ears. First visit to the toilet. Talk in a friendly manner to the patient. Perhaps give them a light tummy massage. The patient could drink a special warm drink, such as hot water with lemon, as recommended in Waerland therapy (treatment of the mind, body and spirit). Then the patient could take a warm shower, followed by a cold rub with a flannel for one minute (starting with the feet and working towards the heart), then rub the body dry. If necessary, a second visit to the toilet (a regular bowel movement is very important). Light gymnastics or massage. After the patient is dressed and if the weather permits, moving about or walking for ten minutes or so in the fresh air.

8 a.m.: Breakfast. If possible, only fruit and herb tea with a little honey. Then relaxation while listening to music. When the weather is bad, light therapy should be given. The patient should lie on a slant board, a few times a day if possible, starting now.

10 a.m.: Outside in the fresh air. Moving about, walking or on an easy chair somewhere sheltered.

11 a.m.: Hydrotherapy (hand or foot baths) or compresses. After this, some relaxation, reading, conversation, drinking some liquid.

12 p.m.: Lunch. Start with a salad if the patient is able to digest this.

1 p.m.: A long rest outside, well covered up. The feet should always be kept warm (if necessary, a foot bath or foot massage should be given). Afterwards, walking or moving about, followed by massage, brush massage, rubbing the patient or other therapy. Make sure the patient drinks enough liquid.

4 p.m.: Hydrotherapy, oil massage. Then some rest and relaxation on the slant board. Drinking some liquid (only if needed or wanted).

5 p.m.: Dinner. Afterwards, relaxation. Early to bed.

During the following weeks, the cleansing therapy should become more and more intensive, until the patient feels much better.

When they learn that a beloved person has Alzheimer's disease, the reaction of relatives is often a feeling of hopelessness and helplessness. One hears constantly that this disease is incurable and that the patient becomes more and more dependent and, in most cases, can no longer be treated at home.

It would make a great difference if people knew that a great deal can in fact be done to hold back for some considerable time the further development of the disease. This knowledge would make it easier for the patient, as well as for the person who takes care of them. One experiences great joy when, now and then, the patient reacts in a positive way, perhaps by smiling again, and the carer feels then that all their work is really worthwhile.

This could all be avoided, though, if we were able to prevent this disease, and this will only be possible when people understand a little more about the connections between living and eating habits, health and disease. Elderly people should stop eating an unbalanced diet, which, unfortunately, most of them do. They should go outside in the fresh air more and regularly exercise their memories. There are many, many ways to keep the body and mind fit – we simply do not usually take the trouble to practise these.

As I have said, in olden times the mentally ill were not seen as incurable. We should learn again to have more faith and not always believe the worst. The human body is, and will always be, something wonderful and we should rediscover how it functions and how we can support nature's endeavours so that healing can be initiated.

In medical circles, for quite a few years now, Alzheimer's disease has been seen as the coming 'plague of the people', or as the 'greatest medical problem' of the future. As this disease afflicts mainly elderly people, the incidence of Alzheimer's will soon rise dramatically owing to the increase in age of the population. Already, millions are being victimised by this illness.

Members of the 'scientific medicine' community are of the opinion that the reason for the enormous increase in this disease is mainly because of the fact that people are living for longer. When a person does not reach a certain age, there is too little time for the symptoms of this disease to present themselves. It is also said that this disease has been occurring for centuries; however, the diagnostic methods needed to recognise the disease have not always been known.

Both arguments are true. The older people get, the greater the possibility that they will develop Alzheimer's disease. In the 60–64 age group, only 1 per cent of people are victims of this disease. For people over 90, this has increased to 30 per cent. Also, it has been confirmed that Alzheimer's disease, or at least very similar problems, has existed for a long time, although it has never affected such numbers as it does today. The medical establishment is very much concerned about this and investment in research has been increased many times over. Everything is being done to hold back this almost explosive development and to find remedies to suppress the symptoms or even make them disappear.

However, 'old age' in itself cannot be considered a disease, otherwise all old people would be ill. But, of course, in most cases, an old body no longer has such a good, functioning defence system as a young one. This is also one of the reasons that people over 90 suffer more from Alzheimer's than people of 60. During the same period of time in which the rate of the disease has been rapidly increasing, there has been a profound and progressive change in our environment and our lifestyle.

Could it be possible that the true and fundamental cause of our so-called, mostly chronic, 'civilisation diseases' lies in our totally changed environment? Could it also be because our organism – and especially our digestive organs – is still the same as it was thousands of years ago, and cannot yet cope with our changed living and eating habits, that so many people are ill?

The human being we know today is not a product of modern times. Over millions of years, its development has been extremely slow. Any small evolution of the human body takes a long, long time and, on the other hand, our environment has (especially lately) been changing at a frantic speed. Although the human brain has been able to adapt quite well to this new and highly technical world, our body cannot cope and is far behind the times. It cannot assimilate most of the new, chemical substances in our nutrition, which do not exist by themselves in nature. Our body cannot digest or use most of these substances and is not capable of fighting the ever-increasing quantities of unnatural toxic material. Also, there is a great loss of energy when such material has to be detoxified or eliminated.

Even very small quantities of some of these chemicals can engender serious and even irreversible damage to the human organism. According to Chemical Abstract Services, a division of the American Chemical Society, nowadays about eight million chemical substances are known. Of this number, about 80,000 are produced commercially. Many of them enter the human body by way of our nutrition or respiration, or through our skin, and in these ways they penetrate our bloodstream. Many of these enter our body on a daily basis. Some of them are incontestably toxic for us. Unfortunately, it is often assumed that because of the small quantities in which they enter our organism, these do not have a toxic effect.

Several years ago, during an exact and detailed examination of Alzheimer's plaques, astrocytes and microglia were discovered. These are precursors of interleukin 6; in other words, they are chemically associated with inflammation. They can recognise foreign matter and prepare this foreign matter for destruction by the immune system of the body. They would normally indicate the presence of bacteria, a virus or toxic substances. During this research programme, it was stated that nothing pointed to a previous bacterial or viral infection. Also, it was said that 'no toxic substances had been discovered'. So, what were these astrocytes and microglia doing in these plaques? It seemed to make no sense . . . As bacteria and viruses have more volume than many toxic substances, we can be quite sure that these have little or nothing to do with Alzheimer's disease. However, in the case of toxic substances, the situation is totally different.

Despite the assertion that toxins were not found, we are not yet able to rule out for sure the presence of extremely small quantities of many toxic substances. From homoeopathy, we have learned how strongly the human organism can react to the smallest quantities of toxic matter, even when no substance whatsoever can be detected and there are only the vibrations of such substances left. From cancer research, we know that the smallest quantities of toxic matter may slowly accumulate in the body cells. Sometimes because of this, but only after many years, cell function can be totally destroyed. We are still too innocent and we do not believe that all these very small quantities of preservatives, insecticides, colourings, cleansing materials, different kinds of sprays and even so-called 'healing remedies' might have consequences to our health. And the extremely dangerous interactions between toxic substances are not even considered, although many dense volumes have already been written about these problems.

In the meantime, much research concerning Alzheimer's disease is being done, mostly with regard to the brain, where the symptoms of the disease can be found. The search is for the cause of the disease, so that, as soon as a 'scapegoat' has been found, an efficient medication can be developed which will remove the symptoms. It seems to have been forgotten that the original causes of most so-called 'civilisation diseases' are multiple. Even if a specific medication could be manufactured, this could never be more than a partial solution and would probably have some dangerous side effects.

About 150 years ago, medical science was changing. 'Symptomatic medicine' – a medicine for emergencies – was being developed. It was very effective and good for treatment of various diseases, in case of accidents and dangerous infections. The suppression of symptoms was the central motive of this kind of medical treatment. Later on, through the development of sulpha drugs and antibiotics, this method was further refined. Symptomatic treatment can sometimes be life-saving and is a great help where accidents, operations and other acute problems are concerned. But this symptomatic medicine is, in itself, only a medicine for emergencies. It has no relation at all to most chronic civilisation diseases and is quite useless with regard to them. It seems amazing that, nevertheless, medical students at university are still being taught the same things.

As a result of technical development, whereby electronics and computer science play an important role, more and more symptoms are being found. Research is being done into the smallest details. Only a few people seem to understand that the ensuing suppression of symptoms – which was so successful a hundred years ago – has nothing to do with real healing.

Science has now progressed into the sphere of gene technology, whereby perhaps now, at last, the real cause – in this case the 'construction error' which causes Alzheimer's disease – may be found. Then Alzheimer's disease can be fought by changing the genes responsible using this amazing new technology. These thoughts do not constitute a mere Utopian dream. It may take 20, 30 or even more years until it will be possible to change those genes. Then, slowly but surely, medicine will be able to root out not only Alzheimer's disease but many other dangerous diseases . . . or perhaps not . . .

In my opinion, the future will be quite different to what is imagined now in many medical circles. There will always be diseases, as what we call 'disease' is part of life. Without it or its symptoms, without those defensive measures our organism takes against threatening dangers, such as toxins, poisons, microbes and many others, our body would soon be destroyed. Maybe one day there will be no Alzheimer's disease, no Down's syndrome or similar diseases. However, instead of these, new diseases – probably even more dangerous and deadly – will come into being. As long as our organism is threatened by all kinds of dangers, nature will always find new ways to defend it. Nature will always be more intelligent than the human being who imagines it to be possible to rule over and control it.

With the help of new and always improving diagnostic procedures like PET (positron emission tomography) and brain mapping, it becomes ever easier to identify changes in the different regions of the brain. In the case of Alzheimer's disease, those regions which have to do with memory and intelligent behaviour become diseased. There, a progressive destruction of brain cells is to be seen. Also, there is a diminished metabolism of glucose. The pattern of blood circulation changes and plaques come into being.

Although many connections are known, there is not yet any certainty as to the cause of Alzheimer's. There is no known cure and the great breakthrough is probably still a long way off. Sometimes it is possible by the use of certain medication to delay further development of the disease. When necessary, physicians and specialists prescribe psychopharma, soothing or invigorating remedies. Some of those are harmless; others, on the contrary, have dangerous side effects, which can often cause irreversible damage.

Alzheimer's disease is not the only disease of the brain which mainly concerns memory and intelligent behaviour. Schizophrenia, hepatitis, encephalopathy, manic depression and similar diseases also show the same kinds of personality changes. Not long ago, mental asylums in the United States were still full of schizophrenic patients. However, about 30 years ago, this situation improved. It was found that many such patients suffered from a lack of very specific substances or from an overload of toxins. Also, in many cases, food allergies were responsible. Sometimes two or three of these factors were responsible for the illness.

Some physicians started to check their patients by using blood and hair analyses in order to find out which heavy metals, insecticides or other toxins were responsible. They also tested sufferers for food allergies. According to their findings, the patients were treated by way of orthomolecular therapy and other specifically targeted medication, which was very successful.

In Britain, Dr Richard Mackarness in particular had much success with the treatment of mentally ill patients. In the United States, Dr Albert Rowe, Dr Herbert Rinkel, Dr Theron Randolph, Dr J.B. Miller, Dr Abram Hoffer, Dr Humphry Osmond and many others put the accent on natural and simple nutrition, and orthomolecular treatment confirmed the value of this method. In Europe, famous personalities like Priessnitz, Schroth, Kneipp, Waerland, Weston Price and physicians like Brauchle, Warburg, Volhard, Wendt, Mommsen, Brucker, Kollath, Kötschau, Bircher-Benner and others showed us in a practical way the importance of a healthy diet and way of living for the maintenance of both physical and mental health.

Unfortunately, this important point of view, which could help millions of patients and their relatives, is understood by only a few physicians, who understand the fact that nowadays we need a completely new attitude to disease. Orthomolecular medicine is as yet not even known to many doctors.

CHAPTER SIX

Boost Your Immune System Naturally

Some time ago, my great friend Dr Hans Moolenburgh and I stood at the bedside of a girl who was being fed intravenously, was wired up to a heart monitor and whose only means of communication was through eye contact. She could neither speak nor move. Fortunately, she was still able to hear and, by blinking her eyelids, she could at least maintain some form of communication. We both witnessed this heartbreaking situation and agreed that if we could only make a breakthrough with the immune system, then we could at least make some headway. The immune system is one of the most complex aspects of our bodies, and it is one which often fails as a result of our lack of precise knowledge on how to tackle it.

We are often reminded that a weak body is constantly vulnerable to bacteria, viruses, fungi and parasites. If our reserves are in peak condition, then we can cope with this, but if they are below par, then those bacteria can multiply rapidly, resulting in the immune system not operating as efficiently as it should. A healthy body has sufficient reserves to fight these bacteria and often balance the system. Scientists have only recently discovered the extent and effectiveness of this self-defensive behaviour by the body. It is amazing to see how macrophages (scavenger cells) work and how our system can be protected by the correct blood cells; on the other hand, we can also see how much damage can be caused when bacteria infiltrate the body. Once this happens, they multiply and leave their toxic material, and unless immediate action is taken, they can harm the body in many different ways.

Although viruses are smaller than bacteria – and both are too small to be seen by the naked eye – they can be even nastier. They cannot multiply until they are inside the body's cells but, once there, they grow rapidly.

Fungi are becoming more common nowadays, and of the hundreds of thousands of different fungi, only a small percentage can make us ill. Our reserves are a great help in this, yet it only takes one of these viruses, fungi or bacteria to cause a great deal of damage. A lot depends on how we live, our dietary management and what the offenders are. A healthy diet is vital, as this will boost the body's immune system whenever it becomes weaker. Good hygiene and a healthy lifestyle are essential. Alfred Vogel, my great friend, spent much of his lifetime talking about the immune system and emphasised the importance of boosting the immune system to make it as strong as possible. I have often said in lectures that we have to be level-headed in our approach to boosting our immune system, as we cannot do this by eating synthetic puddings or a tin of tomato soup that has never seen a tomato. With every second that passes, we lay ourselves open to hundreds of these nasty enemies which can have such a detrimental effect on our system.

I clearly remember the Second World War, when I was a young boy and witnessed at first hand the illnesses and diseases that were around. In the hungry winter of 1944, we were very grateful to the

Red Cross for giving us vitamin C tablets to keep us going until the end of the war. Because food was scarce, people resorted to eating a lot more roughage, as a result of which there were fewer stomach and bowel disorders, or even cases of irritable bowel syndrome, than we currently see. By basically increasing their roughage intake and eating more natural foods, their bodies were actually stronger, unless, of course, there was total starvation.

As a result of having seen thousands of patients during my life, I have investigated the immune system thoroughly, and I have frequently been astonished at the results I have achieved by simply improving a patient's diet. The capabilities of the system never cease to amaze me, and yet we know very little about it. A great friend of mine, one of the most eminent immunologists in Britain, once said to me, 'We may have piles of books on this subject, but yet there are still many unanswered questions.'

So let's have a glance at what the immune system really is. The immune system is the defence mechanism of our body. Part of this is the lymphatic system, which is a net of lymphatic vessels with a similar sort of layout to that of the blood vessels in our organism. From every part of our body, toxic substances are transported via these lymph vessels to the smaller and larger lymph nodes, which are the 'sewage plants' of the body. Bacteria, toxins, alien substances and waste products from the body itself, like dead cells and bacteria, are transported to these detoxification centres.

Some substances, for example those from cow's milk and certain fats, are sent directly from the intestines via the small lymph vessels situated in the intestinal wall to the main centre of the lymphatic defence system, situated in the abdomen. There, and in the other lymph nodes, such as the tonsils and the appendix, the substances mentioned above are cleaned and detoxified. After this, all waste materials which cannot be used are taken up by the venous blood and eliminated. The most important organs through which this elimination of toxins takes place are the skin, the kidneys, the lungs and the intestines. As the greatest dangers that threaten our health develop in the abdomen, most lymphatic vessels and lymph nodes are found there. Here also, a very important substance for our defence, immunoglobulin, is produced. Every second, no matter how slight the danger, millions of defensive cells are used and have to be replaced over and over again. The spleen and the thyroid gland are an important part of this defence system.

Physicians knew hundreds of years ago that there are many interactions between the outer skin and the inner mucus membrane which can be made use of therapeutically. The same is true of the relationship between the skin and the lymphatic system. There are people who have a so-called 'lymphatic constitution'. These people very often become ill when their lymphatic defences have been weakened. They then suffer from health problems, such as the common cold or a sore throat, which are nothing but a simple defence reaction of the body. Such natural reactions always have a purpose, serving to eliminate toxins.

When the health of the organism is at risk, the immune system will automatically react. One can understand this best by observing the simple defensive reactions that happen every day: if dust gets into the nose, we sneeze in order to get rid of it and protect our respiratory tract. Coughing, clearing the throat and sneezing sometimes have a double purpose: they help not only to dispose of dust particles but also to eliminate accumulated mucus. If something gets into the eyes, tears will clean them. If we have eaten some food that does not agree with us, we get diarrhoea or we have to vomit. The main purpose of this is always the cleaning of the organism. Simple health problems will be cured by simple measures. The organism will fight greater health problems by using various stronger defensive measures.

A lymphatic constitution is sometimes hereditary, but it is also possible to acquire such a constitution during the course of life. This can start when one is still young, for example when small children eat too many sweets or drink cow's milk. In this case, the tonsils or the lymph nodes in the neck start to swell as the organism tries to neutralise the toxins. If it is not possible to neutralise all the toxins, the child may get tonsillitis (inflammation of the tonsils). It will depend upon the physician and the parents whether this inflammation is treated in the correct way, by natural means, or whether the child will suffer all its life from lymphatic diseases. An operation on the tonsils or a treatment with antibiotics may have serious consequences, as the tonsils will no longer be able to act as a defensive organism. After some time, other parts of the lymphatic system, such as the bronchial tubes or the mucus membranes of the sinuses, will take over those defensive functions which were formerly the task of the tonsils. If this happens and the person in question eats an unhealthy diet, these secondary defensive systems will also become overstrained. Then, lifelong chronic diseases of the bronchial system and the sinuses, as well as serious diseases of the abdomen, may develop.

Our immune system nowadays has to work non-stop at full power and is constantly overstressed. Cells of the immune system die by the millions and cannot be replaced quickly enough. Innumerable alien substances, which have no place in the human body, prevent normal bodily functions. Any substance entering our digestive tract which cannot be used in some way means needless work for the immune system and a waste of energy.

We live in a world full of harmful substances, toxins, microbes and other tiny creatures, and each day many of these penetrate into our body. Most of the time, such alien elements are rendered harmless by our defensive mechanism and are then eliminated as soon as possible. But until these facts are taught at universities, and as long as all symptoms are suppressed regardless of the consequences, there will be more and more chronic illness in the world.

In studying the immune system, we may amass a lot of information about A lymphocytes, B lymphocytes and T lymphocytes, but we are still faced with one important question: 'How do we look after ourselves?' We need to ask ourselves if we have good dietary management, if we get enough sleep, if we relax enough and if we carry out any detoxification. Vogel's *Detox Box* is of tremendous help in rebuilding one's immunity, and contains beneficial remedies such as *Echinaforce* and *Vital Force* . This programme should be carried out in conjunction with a healthy-eating plan in which, for instance, coffee, tea, alcohol and salt should be avoided and replaced with natural foodstuffs such as Bambu coffee and Herbamare seasoning.

I am always pleased when I see the immune system start to pick up in patients who have been struggling with the problems caused by the post-viral syndrome or myalgic encephalomyelitis (ME). Sometimes, with only a little help, such as introducing a high-quality antioxidant like *Eleutherococcus* (Siberian ginseng), ginseng, ginkgo biloba and some natural vitamins, it is wonderful to see how patients can gain a new lease of life after enduring many years of misery. I remember one young patient who had been suffering with total exhaustion for about five or six years who, following treatment, completely regained his health and told me that life had a purpose again.

Boosting your immune system naturally is a great challenge because your body's immune system can be likened to your own private army for battling disease and defending it against countless intruders. This army is made up of various battalions of different cells with varying and numerous 'army bases' and 'factories' for the supply of all kinds of ammunition. If the 'soldiers' are weak and unhealthy or if the factories are short of raw materials, the army is likely to lose the battle. If the army is in good condition and well equipped, then it will usually be able to fight off diseases. To put it another way, think of your immune system as two opposing armies – one of degenerative cells in combat with one of regenerative cells. If the former appears to be stronger, we must provide the correct materials and weapons for the army of regenerative cells to bolster its defences. It will then have the strength to fight the army of degenerative cells.

We often see this principle at work in the fight against cancer. When people have chemotherapy or radiotherapy, it is not only the degenerative cells that are destroyed but the healthy regenerative cells too. During such highly toxic treatment, it is therefore vital that we boost the regenerative cells by doing everything possible to build up the immune system. An important aspect of that battle is therefore to clear the rubbish out of the system. The ability to clean up the mess – such as the dead invaders, the dead offenders and the chemicals from all the waste material – will help the regenerative system to deal with all the waste that the body can do without.

The fuel has to be of high quality if it is to help protect the body. If it is of poor quality, then dangerous free radicals will be produced. We often see free radicals going haywire and causing havoc, which is sometimes called oxy-stress. This stress mostly affects the state of the immune system and is a major factor in ageing. The most common form of free-radical harm is from poor quality (refined and processed) or rancid oils and fats. The idea of cutting down on the intruders entering the body is not a new one. You have to be aware of this issue and boost your immunity with a simple but nutritious diet. If you can cut out pollutants as much as possible, then you are already making improvements. Drugs and medication can often have an extremely taxing effect on the system. It is therefore a good idea to build up strong walls of defence and to take some remedies specifically for the purpose of boosting the immune system, together with vitamins, minerals, trace elements and *Quick Immune Response,* which will really improve the situation.

So what should we do to help boost or balance the immune system? In a nutshell, first, we need to change to a good, wholesome diet, with proper dietary management; second, we need to undertake regular exercise; third, we need detoxification or an internal cleansing programme; fourth, we need to deal with the stresses that crop up in our lives; and finally, we may need to consider including some supplements.

There is often a misunderstanding about *Echinacea*. Alfred Vogel believed that *Echinacea* was not to be used only to boost the immune system but to balance it, and he used it for that purpose all his life. With autoimmune diseases, one has not only to be careful in boosting the immune system in the short term but also to concentrate on long-term care of the system. *Echinaforce* is an extremely well-balanced product containing *Echinacea purpurea* and can be used indefinitely for this purpose. It will certainly help to build the walls around us when we are attacked daily by viral, bacterial and fungal conditions.

Therapies such as reflexology, aromatherapy and biomagnetic reflex techniques can also be of immense assistance. I have included a diagram here to show these nutritional reflexes and which remedies can have the greatest impact. The nutritional reflexes need to be fed, and therefore dietary management and supplements are necessary.

In my practice, I am aware that life's constant changes often present us with the most unusual situations – such as the number of people dying of metabolic disorders, the lowering of the immune system and the problems that make people vulnerable to attacks by viruses, bacteria and other invaders. I am always amazed at how the body has been created and how the immune system can take over so quickly to defend it when difficulties arise. The biological processes of nature have been so disturbed by man's interference that we often forget what

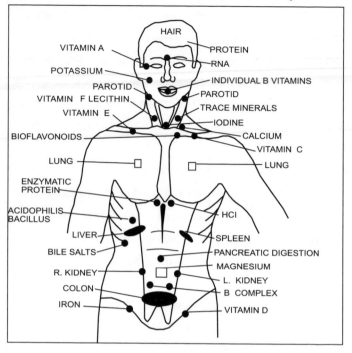

If there is a lack of a particular nutrient, problems
may show up in the relevant reflex zone.

Alfred Vogel always said: 'If we obey the laws of nature, we obey the
laws of Creation.'

In considering the immune system thoroughly, it is amazing what
can be done to build up our resistance, and it never ceases to astonish
me how much our health can be improved by making some minor
adjustments to boost our natural defences. In saying that, however, we
must always remember that prevention is better than cure.

CHAPTER SEVEN

Easy Ways to Relieve Stress and How to Relax

We all speak so glibly about stress and probably don't realise the effects that it has on our health. Not only can anxiety and tension be very damaging at the time we are experiencing them but they can also cause problems further down the line, so we must learn how to deal with this problem before it escalates into something more serious in later life.

One Christmas Day, my eldest granddaughter, who was then in her second year at university, studying medicine, asked me to go with her to visit a well-known and well-loved medical professor, whom I have known personally for many years. They had become quite friendly and she often talked to him. When we visited this gentleman, who is now elderly, I could see he was under a lot of stress. On the one hand, life had been good to him, but on the other hand, he had to cope with many stressful situations, not only when he had lost loved ones but also later on in his life, when he was faced with other worries. The stress he had endured hadn't been taken care of at the time and this had resulted in him now being nervous and upset. I talked to him for a little while about the good parts of his life, and because I knew he was loved by his students, I also made reference to all the good he had done. I urged him to try to relax as much as possible and to enjoy himself as best he could in his advanced age. When we left him, I listened proudly as my granddaughter spoke with a great deal of wisdom. As we discussed stress, we agreed how important it is to get to grips with it while we are still able and before it leads to long-term health complications. As one becomes older, it is not as easy to recognise the signs of stress and nervous conditions as it is when one is younger. It is therefore necessary that we understand what stress is all about. As I have said, we talk so flippantly about it and yet it can cause so many serious health problems.

I remember a patient who was a famous musician and who, in later life, became an equally famous artist. I can still vividly recall him coming to see me. He was extremely depressed because he had lost the tips of two fingers following an infection, which had led to difficulties in him playing the violin. We talked for a long time. I felt sorry that he was in such a distressed state and I could see that he was actually suicidal. I realised that he needed a lot of understanding to help him deal with this problem. I phoned his wife when he left me and asked her to keep an eye on him. When she said that she too felt he was suicidal, that made me even more determined to help him overcome his despair. We had talked about our mutual interest in sailing, and I had asked him if he would like to come out with me. It was arranged that we would go the following day. As we talked, I said that I understood his need to express his emotions through his music – his every thought, every frustration and every moment of happiness – but suggested that he could perhaps capture these sentiments just as deeply (if not more so) through painting. When he replied that he couldn't even draw, I urged him to try and, as an incentive, I bought him some paints, a piece of canvas, a few brushes and some pencils. I asked him to start drawing and see what happened.

To cut a long story short, he took great pleasure in it and his very first painting has been hanging in the hall of my main clinic at Auchenkyle all these years. It wasn't until he started painting that he realised he could indeed convey his thoughts onto the canvas. He took a very strong interest in it and became even more famous as an artist than he was as a musician – his paintings are still sold for huge sums of money today. In one fell swoop, he was able to get rid of all the stress from his life and transmit the true value of his thoughts into his paintings.

It is not always easy to overcome stress, yet it is essential that we do, for it is very dangerous. One must not forget that a great many degenerative diseases are a result of stress. As a member of the Cancer Control Society in the United States, I can honestly say that, during my lifetime, I have seen many cancer cases that have resulted from stress. It attacks the sufferer not only emotionally and mentally but also physically.

This reminds me of a famous singer whom I recognised immediately when she walked into my clinic in Harley Street. I could see the stress on her face as she told me that her singing had gone downhill. She had no idea what was wrong and was naturally very worried. As she spoke to me, I noticed straight away that her jaw was out of place, which can easily happen in stressful situations or sometimes even as a result of visiting the dentist. If a dentist puts too much pressure on a problematic tooth, for example, the jaw can easily come out of place. This can affect the temporal mandible joint and the hyoid bone, which has an influence on the voice. In fact, this woman confirmed that she had indeed recently attended the dentist. I managed to adjust her jaw in seconds and was able to correct the situation. A short time later, she telephoned me to say that her singing had improved and that her jaw was much better. Nowadays, her voice is better than ever.

Making an adjustment like this is an easy way to release stress and also to nip a problem in the bud.

We need to accept that stress is unavoidable in this day and age and that therefore we must learn how to deal with it, preferably before it reaches a level at which it could be really damaging. We have to try to eradicate it from our lives before it escalates into something more serious. I will admit that my first book, *Stress and Nervous Disorders,* was quite poorly written. My knowledge of the English language was not very good at that time. And yet that book has sold more copies than any of the other 40-plus books I have written. I have often been intrigued as to why and have reached the conclusion that because this is a massive problem which affects individuals from all walks of life, many people want to read all about it, which is a responsible thing to do.

Since writing that book, I have had several experiences in my own life which have resulted in my gaining a deeper awareness of stress, allowing me to better understand my patients' problems. As a child growing up during the Second World War, I could cope with the stress when the Germans tried to shoot us. I could handle the problems of adolescence and the anxieties that cropped up during my student days, and nowadays I can deal with the enormous stresses I have with patients who don't respond the way I want. What I cannot cope with, however, is injustice. One particular incident in my life which I found extremely difficult to handle and which upset me greatly was when jealous colleagues conspired against me. This conspiracy led to a lot of injustice and the strain attacked my system, particularly emotionally. As the heart controls the emotions, that specific problem robbed me of an extremely healthy heart and left me with a diseased heart. I was reminded once more of how traumas can cause severe problems.

Life expectancy is much longer nowadays, and this is another reason why we must be careful not to let stress take its toll on our health. I think about such people as the novelist Iris Murdoch. A film released in 2002 told the story of her life and its deterioration due to Alzheimer's disease. It is essential that we learn to understand about stress and emotion and to pay great attention to stress, particularly when overworked. I once visited an eminent doctor who was admired by everyone. What a brilliant brain he had during his working life! He was extremely conscientious but due to worries about his children and taking his work very seriously (something which can be very rewarding under the right conditions, of course), it all sadly became too much for him. When I visited him in a psychiatric institution, I was shocked to see such a decline in this great man. He did not know where he was or what he did. I really wept when I left him, wondering how this brilliant brain could end up like this. No one in his family had this illness – it could perhaps be genetic, nobody knows. However, one reason may possibly have been due to the kind of life he led.

It is advisable to deal with health issues while we are still fit and able, and to take whatever steps necessary to try to prevent such degenerative diseases arising as we become older. As I have said previously, prevention is better than cure, and we have to learn the art of relaxation, which I shall go into later.

STRESS – A DISEASE OF MODERN TIMES

Let's have a look at what stress really is. Evidence is growing that stress lies at the core of most physical, mental and social problems of our time. Stress is a part of life. We all need a certain amount in order to improve and develop our mental and physical potential. The right amount of stress can be a challenge; life without stress would be extremely dull. However, in our time, we suffer from far too much stress. There is too much noise, and there are too many people and far too many toxins in our food, in the water, in the soil and in the air around us. Also, the aggressive and egotistical behaviour of many people towards their fellow human beings is a very serious cause of stress. Stress is a normal reaction to changes in our daily life. It can be physical, mental or both, and as long as a particular form of stress does not last too long, it can be a positive experience. When it is of long duration, though, this kind of stress can cause not only physical diseases, like high blood pressure and gastric and duodenal ulcers, but also various kinds of mental problems and diseases.

From its earliest beginnings, human life was often endangered, and adrenalin made people aware of these dangers and prepared the body, as well as the mind, for fight or flight. These reactions are still the same today, even when the stress only exists in our imagination. Of course, the stress factor not only affects us by an invariable breakdown of tissue but also has a terrific impact on the heart. Alfred Vogel said that the ever-increasing pace that characterises our modern life is one of the worst poisons for our heart. Even though, for the most part, individual productivity has not exceeded that of former times, it has become the custom to cram too many activities, especially those connected with our job, into a short space of time. Our workaholic culture means that we have hardly any time away from our desks, and the free time we do have is hardly ever used in a wholesome recreational or relaxing way such as pursuing a hobby – say, working on an arts and crafts project, listening to good music or acquiring more knowledge through a study course. Instead, we continue at the same hectic pace we keep up for work and seem to find enjoyment at weekends in the midst of the mad world of crowded motorways.

No wonder the result is a state of complete exhaustion instead of recuperation from the week's work. Driving at high speed creates anxiety and inner tension, and affects the heart like a poison. Not only is the speed of the drive harmful but the exhaust fumes are dangerous to the heart and blood vessels, too. How much more sensible it would be to take a short, leisurely ride to a nearby forest or the hills, get out of the car and go for a relaxing walk or hike. This kind of exercise would be invigorating for the blood vessels and, of course, the heart. The time spent in a clean environment would then permit us to return to work and our duties on Monday morning refreshed and relaxed, instead of tense and irritable as is so often the case when we misuse our leisure time.

A similar tendency that should also be mentioned here is that of senselessly abusing our energies by allowing too little time to get to our place of work. We should always leave the house early enough that it is not necessary to make a dash for the bus or train. Even a short run with a briefcase or bag can be more taxing on the heart than most people realise. Obese people should be especially careful and remember the warning contained in the old proverb 'Haste makes waste'. It has become a habit with many to rush around as if they have no time to lose, even though the time gained may be wasted later on in an idle telephone conversation or an insignificant chat with a neighbour. This is really most unwise, for the heart is not like a modern engine that can be accelerated from a standing start to 60 mph in seconds. The heart cannot be driven at top speed without suffering some damage. Even young people who participate in over-strenuous sporting activities can develop dilation of the heart or other heart trouble. Sadly, modern athletic competition no longer attaches importance to purity and style of performance but requires the athlete to give their all, and it is exactly this excessive speed, measured in split seconds, that is dangerous. The excesses will act like poison to the heart, particularly for those athletes who are not in constant training. More often than not, the damage is permanent.

Even those who manage to escape the long working week typical in Britain by working part-time or on flexitime do not necessarily escape stress. The shorter working week is also detrimental to the heart, since the work must be done faster if the number of working days is reduced without a proportionate reduction in the workload. The heart would only benefit from such an arrangement if a more sensible pace of work could be maintained. If a shorter working week depends on increased speed to produce the same results, the health of employee and employer alike will suffer.

Leisure, a cosy home atmosphere, tranquillity and contemplation, a period of relaxation at the end of a working day – these are things that will soon only be known from reading descriptions of the past. Even at mealtimes, modern man is in the grip of a restlessness connected with his busy schedule. Mind you, the body cannot stand this pace of life for ever and the natural outcome is seen in the constant increase in gastric disturbances. We should not be in a hurry when we sit down to eat. In fact, we should rest for a few minutes beforehand and then enjoy our meal with a calm mind and a healthy appetite. Most gastric problems will disappear if we make an effort to be relaxed at mealtimes, eat slowly and chew the food thoroughly. It will then be better assimilated and cause fewer disturbances in the intestines. Also, when chewing thoroughly, you will be less tempted to eat too much, giving you a chance to combat excess weight more effectively. It is an undeniable fact that in the Western world, more people become sick and die as a result of overeating than because of going hungry. We would do well, therefore, to reduce our intake of food and so benefit our health.

Not only can stress have a direct damaging effect on our health, it can also be the cause of psychosomatic illness. Psychosomatic disease today, with world and national unrest, is on the increase and, in many cases, the psychosomatic patient can, and indeed does, develop the symptoms of the disease which they believe they have – for instance, rheumatism, backache, cramps, asthma, heart trouble, gastrointestinal problems, genito-urinary disease, glandular dysfunction, in fact, disease of any part of the body – even though all the physical tests of their tissues are found to be normal. Psychiatry labels this physiological phenomenon as 'escapism', or an effort on the part of the mind to evade the negative impulses which bombard it from the outside.

What does this prove? It proves that the orthodox treatment meted out today can be useless. The best we can say of it is that it is palliative. It does not strike at the primary cause of the complaint and the patient is forced to come back time and time again. You may treat the symptoms of an illness, but if you do not look at the patient's environment, heredity and the day-to-day emotional stress they may be undergoing, it will not help.

CRANIAL STRESS RESPONSE

One of the greatest causes of disease today is tension due to emotional stress, and if we are to arrive at any understanding of it, we must examine the neuro-endocrine functions which produce this. It is unbelievable how many people there are who are asking for advice on how to combat tensions and how few healers there are available who are really qualified and understand the biological basis of tension. Looking back at the many books on the subject of stress and tension, all that these writings seem to have accomplished is to have emphasised its unquestionable importance. Very little that is concrete has been researched or offered for the relief of these stresses and tensions.

It is vital that one should first understand the cause or causes of disease if one is to be in a position to offer any rational treatment. When it comes down to it, one realises that although there are supposedly many diseases, really these are just names for the various symptoms that may be prominent. Apart from accident or trauma, there is only one cause of disease and that is congestion – for example, congestion of the lymphatic system. Try always to keep this in mind and do not let the many names for symptoms add to the confusion.

To really get to grips with stress or tension (congestion), we must understand the nerve-endocrine functions that create it. Many credit the nerves with being the cause of all tension; others attribute it to dysfunction of the endocrine glands, stating that these have a profound influence on the emotions. This is over-simplifying the issue. The combined effect of the nerves and the glands is a physiological phenomenon that is of utmost importance and should be examined in detail to enable us to see how emotional imbalance and stress can be the cause of disease.

One factor is the excretion of sympathin by the terminal endings of the sympathetic nerve. This is more or less identical in nature to the adrenalin released by the adrenal glands. Excitation is the primary cause for the release of these secretions. There is also a reciprocal action between the two, so that every time adrenalin is released, sympathin is too, and vice versa. When we visualise that, on average, there are 62,000 miles of blood vessels, all interlaced with nerve fibres, we can see that this dual sympathin/adrenalin release under acute or chronic stress conditions can produce a terrific shock syndrome and, in some extreme instances, can cause death where the initial stimulation was brought on by acute fear or terror. It must be realised that the release of these substances sets up a vicious cycle wherein tensions tend to create more tensions. Over-excitation, due to daily stress, environment and so on, tends to be self-perpetuating, causing actual tissue change and, in time, death.

Another factor in the problem of emotional stress is organ or gland disturbance, and the relationship between the emotions and both of these.

Fortunately, we can identify all these conditions clinically and eradicate them in between one and three cranial massage treatments with the knowledge we have at our disposal. The reaction is usually positive after the first treatment and the changes that take place in the vascular, endocrine and emotional systems are more than gratifying.

The shock effect of post-surgical and old traumatic cases is cumulative in nature, resisting every known form of therapy until released. Therefore, shock release is a must in the initial treatment stage of many patients.

A great deal of research has been undertaken in the field of neurodynamics, particularly into the emotional areas of the brain. This has been approached from many different standpoints and using a variety of methods, including the application of carbon dioxide, with considerable success. But the main interest has been centred on the control of the blood supply to the various emotional centres of the brain. There are great possibilities in this area. Simple electrical instruments have verified this in showing the amount of blood present in various areas of the brain. Stress on the hormonal system can be greatly relieved nowadays with remedies such as *Menosan* (*Salvia*), Alfred Vogel's great medicine, which can be used for menopausal stress as well. Also available is a great remedy called *Phytogen,* which contains flax-seed oil. These are both of tremendous help in relieving hormonal stress.

The condition of the endocrine, or body energy, balance is important when it comes to relieving stress. The cranial massage described at the end of Chapter Three can be very helpful, as can aromatherapy, acupuncture and reflexology, the last of which I will go into in more detail here.

Body Energy Balance – Touch Method

To *stimulate* the energies in the body, the method used is similar to charging the human battery. The positive (right) hand is always applied to the positive (right) side, i.e. right hand on right side (front of body) and right hand on positive left (back of the body). Also the negative (left) hand is applied to the negative (left) side, i.e. the left side of the front of the body and the right side of the back.

To *sedate* the energies, the contact must be made to continue the flow of energies – positive (right) hand on negative (left) front of body or on the negative (right) on the back. Also the negative (left) hand is applied to the positive (right) side of the front of the body and to the positive (left) side of the back of the body.

Too much pressure should never be applied. The therapist should *not* rub or massage the area – just hold it firmly with the whole hand or with the thumb of the hand, as required.

This method utilises the electrical energy flow by touch. This energy is generated by the healer applying the treatment. The contact between persons penetrates through the skin and circulates in the patient's body – it penetrates deeper and deeper until it reaches the bone structure and then it reverses its journey back to the point of contact.

The length of each area of treatment can vary from two to five minutes. The total of each treatment on various areas should not exceed 30 minutes at any one sitting. The practitioner's energies must not be allowed to fatigue.

If you undergo this method of laying on of hands, you will come to observe that, at times, the practitioner puts the right hand on the left side and the left hand on the right side. To add to this, when the healer is giving a set treatment, they should replenish the patient's body energy with their own energy by placing their right hand on the patient's right hand and their left hand on the patient's left hand. In this way, the patient's own body energy is enhanced by the healer's body energy. This is very powerful in helping the sick.

There is no doubt that these energies do exist and do work to heal every organ, tissue, muscle, bone and so on as a direct or indirect result of contact with the surface area of the human body. This was found to be so by the ancient Chinese 2,000 years ago – today, scientists are realising the truth of the matter.

It is logical when one understands the workings of the sympathetic nerves and the parasympathetic nerves which supply the bones, muscles, blood and so on with a strong energy to contract and expand. This is the secret of life – where there is no movement, there is no life. It has been tested, ascertained and proved that many nerve centres exist on the surface of the skin and it is really through these centres that one endeavours to heal by stimulating or sedating the inherent universal energies.

Body Energy Balance – the Feet

The endocrine zones on the foot are clearly marked on the diagram over the page. When giving a treatment, a practitioner will hold these zones with one hand and firmly press on them. The zones on the left foot are treated with the right hand (as the left foot is negative and the right hand is positive). The left hand can then contact the zones on the patient's cranium and this will complete the energy circuit. Similarly, the zones on the right foot are held with the left hand while the right hand is used on the cranial endocrine zones.

The secret of this endocrine balance is bringing into play the triune qualities of body energy – positive, negative and neutral. The thumb of each hand should be used for the contact – the thumb is the neuter energy pole. This simple but very deep-acting endocrine balance treatment can help anyone. The zones on the foot allow the practitioner to reach the all-important centres of life and maintain the balance of body energy.

It can be said to be true that the conscientious application of this simple technique can bring miraculous relief from harmful tensions and also from psychosomatic factors. Glandular or endocrine massage will rid you of a feeling of exhaustion.

Stress – the Feet

One can see how much can be done to the feet to aid relaxation and regain a lot of energy. The methods of working on the feet practised in

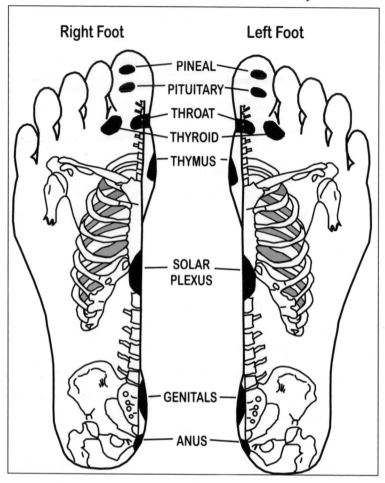

Right Foot   Left Foot

PINEAL
PITUITARY
THROAT
THYROID
THYMUS

SOLAR
PLEXUS

GENITALS

ANUS

The endocrine reflex zones of the feet

Oriental medicine are totally different from those written about by Western practitioners. Many techniques have been used to relieve pain, suffering and stress, but none as valuable as relief through the traditional Chinese practice of reflexology. Many stubborn cases have found relief through foot-reflex release – it is true, though some may find it hard to believe.

Each part of the body that is in touch with the outside world has its own set of reflexes, which reflect every part of our bodies and minds. It is plain if we look at ourselves in daily life – our feet communicate with the earth we stand on and our heads with the heavens above.

There are various fantastic books on foot and hand reflexes. More information on this subject is contained in my book *Body Energy*.

It has been my experience that I have much better results by first examining the feet, then adjusting them and finally massaging them. One of the simple adjustments I use is as follows. The cuboid is the cornerstone of the Gothic arch of the foot. To adjust, I make a paddle contact with the left hand at the back of the tuberosity of the fifth metatarsal. The right hand is positioned over the opposite side of the foot with the thumb under the arch. Then both elbows are brought up and away with a snap. In my practice, it has been found that if one adjusts the cuboids, it is not necessary to spend time on the other bones that make up the foot.

Before reflex massage is carried out, it is a good idea to make sure the feet are healthy and in good condition. The commonest forms of foot complaint are:

Calluses and hard corns. These are build-ups of dead skin, and anybody can trim them painlessly. Simple remedies can be helpful too, but Dr Alexander Hersh notes that older persons, diabetics, those suffering from arthritis, peripheral vascular disorders or others who experience difficulty in treating their own corns and calluses should seek professional help.

Soft corns. These arise between the toes, resulting from local bone pressure. They represent a hazard if self-doctored and should be treated professionally.

Pain in the ball of the foot. This can be caused by several factors: a neuroma (an enlargement of nerve fibres), excessively high arches, hammer toes or an excessively shortened Achilles tendon. Sufferers should seek professional guidance for proper treatment.

Itching, rash or pimples. These are skin problems that should be treated by those in the profession who have dermatological expertise, but, as a temporary measure, the use of a skin-conditioning supplement can be very helpful.

Ingrown toenails. These can be caused by poorly fitting shoes or socks, deformed nails or improper pedicure. The proper way to cut one's toenails is straight across, rather than in a rounded shape. If, for some reason, a nail continues to grow into the toe, or the person (because of age or disability) can't cut their nails properly, they should get a professional pedicure from a podiatrist.

Bunions. This condition results when the big toe drifts in the direction of the other toes, sometimes overlapping the second toe, and the head of the first metatarsal bone becomes enlarged. A painful condition, it can be caused by wearing narrow, pointed shoes, or by hereditary factors. It should never be self-treated. Professional help should always be sought.

Flat feet. While most parents tend to mistake a normal pad of fat in their children's feet for flat-footedness, this condition does exist in certain youngsters and is generally hereditary. In mild cases, those afflicted can get along on well-constructed shoes and/or a plastic arch support. Severe cases require professional care and possibly corrective shoes.

Once you have sorted out any foot ailments and the cuboids have been examined and treated where necessary, the feet will be ready for reflex massage. It has been my experience that various ailments respond to this type of treatment with miraculous results.

There is a rule concerning the three main approaches that should be used towards any problem in life. The hips govern the 'going' principle, the shoulders the 'doing' principle and the head the 'thinking' principle. The diaphragm controls the thymus and lung area, which defines the quality of our life. An old Indian saying is as follows: 'All body fluids correspond to the emotional principle, soft tissue to the mental principle, and hard tissue to the spiritual principle.'

I have found that most heart cases have trouble in the solar plexus area. Even diabetes has a definite reference to the solar plexus. The solar plexus is important because this is the centre of the hormonal system. It has a very disturbing effect when it is in a state of tension. Stress always shows in the feet, like a telephone switchboard – when the light comes on it shows which line is being called. It isn't really the light which is significant, but the circuit which creates it. The cause must be treated before the symptom will be relieved. The reflex zones of the feet are shown in the diagrams on pp. 194–5.

The therapist must make a study of the arches in the feet: a fallen, longitudinal arch reflects back to the solar plexus; the metatarsal arch reflects the quality of the nervous system; while nail defects, corns and calluses usually indicate a condition of stress.

The treatment of these stress areas is easily carried out with the side of the thumb. The areas should not be massaged. An inhibitory movement is made and held for a few seconds – this affects the lymphatic system in the area being treated.

I should add that the following complaints can be helped wonderfully by relieving the corresponding stress areas in the human foot:

Allergies: the solar plexus area
Apoplexy: work should be done on the same side as the brain area
Arthritis: the solar plexus, kidneys and colon areas
Asthma: the lymphatic zones, the endocrine zones and the ileocaecal areas

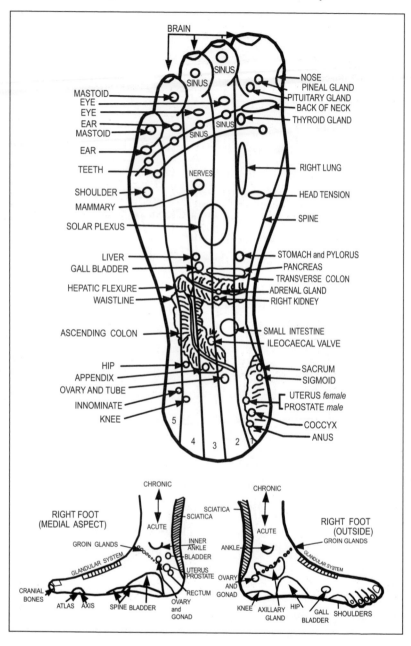

Atlas and axis: this can be loosened by rotation of both big toes

Coronary: the cervical area

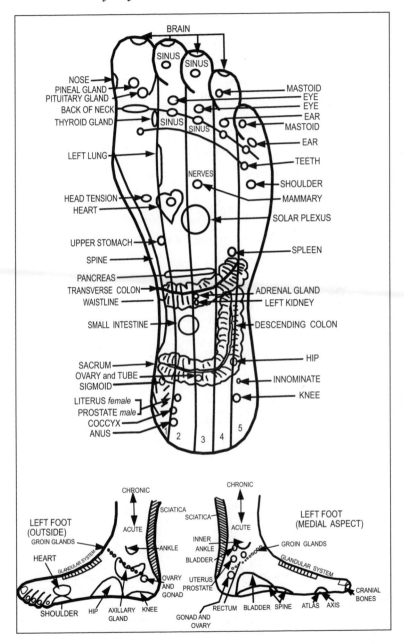

Endocrine gland problems: all the endocrine zones should be treated if any one of the glands is tender

Enuresis: the solar plexus, the bladder (kidneys and the endocrine zones)

Epilepsy: the endocrines, the colon and the ileocaecal areas

Hips: the shoulder joint on the corresponding side should be treated, also around onto the ankle

Hyper- and hypotension: the head zones; could be due to the prostate (kidneys or solar plexus areas). Treat accordingly.

Insomnia: the suprarenals and solar plexus area (efficacious in cases of extreme tiredness)

Knees: the elbow joints, also the sacral area of the foot

Muscle tone: to increase, the suprarenals should be treated

Nerve tension: the lymphatic and solar plexus areas, the endocrine zones

Sinuses: the ileocaecal valve area, the sinus areas of the feet

Tonsillitis: the lymphatic drainage area and outer ankles

Varicose veins: the colon area; the veins themselves should not be touched

It has often been found that kidney and prostate trouble can be the underlying cause of rheumatic pain. In migraine, it would be good to look at the pituitary and gall bladder areas on the feet.

Remember that the principle of foot compression used here should not be confused with the ordinary form of massage. A totally different method is involved; the foot should not be stroked but an applied pressure should be employed with the thumb. The simplicity of this method should command your attention. The more simple it is, the more effective the results.

Here are a few more pieces of information regarding reflex massage:

- In **anaemia**, the spleen is involved, so that area of the foot should be treated (pernicious anaemia is slower to respond).

- The **spleen** also has an effect on the large and small intestines and can, at times, cause a disturbance in the colon.

- Always remember that if pain increases after a foot reflex treatment, it is a sign that some pathological symptoms may be involved in the reflex zones.

- Patients with **arthritis** should have the area of the feet directly connected or reflexed by having the stomach and intestinal zone firmly massaged.

- **Hay fever** as well as **sinus** conditions can be attacked by working on the feet around the area of the big toe.

- The glandular areas should be massaged if you want to rid yourself of **exhaustion**. The massage should start with the pineal and pituitary areas, working down the feet.

- **Depression** is connected with body fatigue and will also respond to endocrine or glandular zone massage.

- **Lack of energy** can be helped with a liver reflex massage of the feet (this should be done cautiously and gently).

It is very interesting to see that the operation of the nervous system can be influenced so much by these particular treatments.

As I have said, people talk glibly about tension. They must be thinking only of mental tension, which in itself is serious enough. Tension, inner conflict, emotional upsets – these are what cause most functional disease, and these factors, when persistent, actually precipitate soluble calcium from the bloodstream into the joints. Mind has thus become matter. The result can be arthritis, rheumatism or lumbago. This might be called the negative miracle. The positive miracle is to supplant tension and worry with such tendencies as joy, happiness and such ideal conditions for survival.

Muscular tension can be produced by cold weather (in which we automatically tense ourselves) or by emotional stimuli such as worry, fear and anxiety. A muscle is capable of contraction and relaxation. In muscular spasm, the blood is squeezed out of the spastic muscle, oxygen cannot get to the tissues and nature then gives its warning – pain.

Contraction of muscle is due to impulses passing via a spinal nerve trunk to the nerve endings of the muscle. In a normal person, this contraction, followed by relaxation – usually due to exercise – improves the metabolism and also increases the circulation of the blood which flows through the muscle, and thus the muscle is strengthened. When the nerves, through disease or injury, are no longer able to conduct these nerve impulses, in most cases, muscle contraction becomes impossible. When a muscle remains contracted, on the other hand – due to spasm, for instance – the results are fatigue, pain and other harmful effects. The supply of oxygen is cut off, and the blood and lymph are squeezed out of the tissues affected. This kind of tension in the muscles can lead to diseases such as fibrositis and neuritis.

It is not generally known that asthma is also due to a spasm which, when the lungs are about to evacuate the air inhaled, prevents expiration or breathing out by dilating the alveoli of the lungs and contracting the bronchial tubes. This complaint can make the life of the sufferer a real martyrdom. Angina pectoris is essentially also caused by a spasm, one which obstructs the coronary arteries (the arteries which convey nutrients and oxygen to the cardiac muscles) so that the blood can no longer reach the tissues of the body.

So we can see that it is vital that we are able to really relax. Once a few relaxation methods have been mastered, they will become an easy and quick routine to relieve stress and tension. If you put in a little effort, relaxation will give you complete control over the stress that might invade your life, or that has been present for a long time.

I have written many books on the subject of relaxation. One can relax through swimming, cycling, walking, yoga, aerobics, golf, the Alexander technique or many other activities and therapies that I could list. It is not my intention to write about various forms of relaxation here. My main aim is that we understand, with our busy daily schedules, that we should relax more often. We need to sit down and perhaps meditate or at least ensure that the body gets a chance to recover from our daily stresses.

Apart from sleep, the body requires a further form of relaxation. Often a workaholic will say that their job is their relaxation, because they enjoy it, it is like a hobby. Nevertheless, they forget that there is a slow and gradual build-up of tension within the body, and many illnesses can result from stress when the body does not receive the opportunity to relax. I have seen many cancer patients who have become the victims of stressful situations. Cells recovering from cancer are very much like brain cells – they require rest and meditation. When I look at my old friends who are well over 100 years of age, I am amazed at how relaxed and balanced they are in their approach to life. This reinforces my belief that it is of the utmost importance to find the correct balance, knowing when to stop and give the body a rest.

Stress and disease are common at the beginning of this new millennium. I often recall that, according to Dr Hans Selye, the Viennese endocrinologist whose research into stress became world renowned in the middle of the last century, we all need a measure of stress. Normal stress is a challenge, which strengthens the body's own defences. However, abnormal stress, from which millions of people in the industrial countries suffer, can overtax us physically as well as mentally. Health and illness are based on very specific natural laws, which must always be observed. These laws concern the constant changes of being awake and asleep, day and night, work and relaxation, happiness and sadness, and so on. In the past, people were obliged to go early to bed and get up early. In those times, daily life depended on daylight, as candles were expensive. In our time, there are many people who do not go to sleep before midnight, or even later. As our organism still reacts to natural sources of light, this habit usually has a negative effect on the nervous system.

In our industrial countries, there are millions of people who work only in order to earn the money they need for their livelihood. They do not care for the work as such and this can be considered a very negative stress factor. Unfortunately, although most people now earn much more than ever before, this does not improve their health. Apart from normal daily expenses, what do people do with their money? They often buy things which they like but do not really need. By making things their possessions, they try to build up their 'image'. This means they want to impress friends and neighbours, to prove they are doing well, according to the principle that people who have many possessions are very clever and should be admired. The more primitive a person is the more they want to possess and to buy. Therefore, they always need more money and have to work harder. In this way, countless people get into an unheeded and constant stress situation.

People who work should also relax. However, many people think that relaxation equates with modern entertainments like television, visiting nightclubs or holidays, which are often far too strenuous and bring no true relaxation. People eat and drink too much and many of them try to forget their problems through intoxicating amusement. This frequently brings more disadvantages than advantages. One has only to think about bad television programmes or about modern so-called sports, which deal more with sensation and business than with real sport. In order not to lose the initial excitement, the different stimuli have to be increased all the time. The thrill of today becomes the boredom of tomorrow and we hardly know any satisfaction.

Real relaxation does not seem to exist any more. Delight arising from beautiful things and the adventure of living is known only to a few. Although young people still spend some of their time in the fresh air, often the oxygen inhaled during the day will be wasted in nightclubs and sometimes hearing will be harmed irreparably. In the same way, the businessman tries to compensate for unhealthy living habits, such as a stressful and sedentary lifestyle and many business dinners, by going jogging or taking up some other weekend sport, which will hardly make him healthy.

Many refugees and immigrants from, for example, Eastern Europe or the developing world become ill because of fear, stress and homesickness. There is another reason for their susceptibility to illness: the unusual food. When observing our fellow human beings at the supermarket, we may see that these newcomers often load up their shopping trolleys with a great amount of food. As soon as these people earn more money than they were used to, most of their earnings will be used to buy food. This stems partly from an unconscious fear of going hungry and also from the fact that many people still think that to eat great quantities of food improves health. It is a fact that carbohydrates often give a sense of security, safety and consolation. For these people, quantity is very important and they do not know anything about the quality of the unfamiliar products they buy – everything looks so nice – so that many of them become not only mentally but also physically ill. The stress of foreign food has been added to their mental stress. Who will help these people?

People are often frightened and usually their fears are totally unfounded. Everybody should examine their fears and try to imagine what would happen if what they fear most really happened. The self-help expert Dale Carnegie wrote that things hardly ever become as bad as we fear. In most cases, this kind of anxiety brings about unheeded stress, which only harms us.

Excess stress can result in a build-up of toxicity, which can lead to many problems. We only need to look at irritable bowel syndrome, which is basically the result of a combination of an incorrect diet and stress. These factors result in a toxic condition being formed in the bowel. The bowel reacts against this and, if we do not address the warning, further problems can occur. Why not look at changing the diet or try taking a good antioxidant? Alternatively, taking remedies such as *Iberogast* and *Tormentil Complex* can quickly resolve the situation. In addition, do not forget that there are many non-addictive preparations that can be taken to eliminate extra stress or nervous anxiety, or ease the unconscious turmoil that invites and causes the onset of health problems and disease.

When stress is not severe and lasts only for a short time, everything soon returns to normal and we recover quickly. However, when stress is more severe and lasts for a long time, we try to adapt to the new situation, assuming that we can resist the effects of stress indefinitely. Therein lies the danger. Believing that we are immune to the effects of stress, we typically fail to do anything about it. If high levels of stress are allowed to continue, exhaustion begins and our self-defence mechanism cannot cope with the stress any more. By and by, the body's reserves succumb and finally the whole organism breaks down. At this point, serious physical and mental diseases may develop. By learning relaxation and stress-management techniques, it is possible to improve your overall health and change many negative, destructive thoughts into positive, healing reactions.

Dr Selye also made the observation that the hormonal changes which take place as soon as a person is confronted with a stressful situation are due, at least partly, to the chemical make-up of each individual. He was convinced that during stress the body loses its chemical balance and that this could be put right by chemical intervention. Although many scientists did not agree with his ideas, pharmaceutical companies smelled big business and billions of dollars were, and still are, made selling mind-changing medication. However, such medication often does more harm than good, because when stress is suppressed by the use of strong medication, many patients lose their former personality.

Always in a hurry to suppress symptoms and make money, the pharmaceutical industry and the medical establishment ignored one of the most important natural laws. This law, which predominates in all natural processes, decrees that only the weakest stimuli can restore health and well-being, that stronger stimuli will do harm and that the strongest stimuli always destroy. Classical medicine seems to have a preference for strong medication, the stronger and more concentrated the better, thereby often destroying the extremely sensitive natural symbiosis, the ecosystem of our brain and nerve centres. As long as modern medicine does not understand this, its remedies will always harm the patient in the long run. The only remedies I recommend in the case of too much stress are homoeopathic and other natural remedies.

Some people can cope much better with physical and mental stress than others; it depends on our personality, our way of life, our medical history and many other factors. Whenever there is stress, we should try to get rid of it as soon as possible and find a way of adjusting our lives in order to lose our nervous tension.

WHAT STRESS MEANS TO BABIES AND SMALL CHILDREN

Some babies are quiet and seldom cry. Other babies cry very often indeed and once in a while even seem to be inconsolable. A baby is a very sensitive little creature and, when its parents are under severe stress, it will react accordingly. A baby can also be stressed when it is dressed too warmly, when there is too much noise, when it feels pain and, above all, when its tummy hurts and its formula is wrong. A baby can become irritable and nervous, suffer from sleeplessness and even become very angry when something is bothering it too much. Babies need lots of love and affection.

Baby formulas, and indeed the nutrition given to children of any age group, are sometimes lacking in many of the most needed nutrients. Sweet foods are often low in vitamins and minerals and high in saturated fats. Sugar becomes a serious problem when sweets, cakes and other snack foods replace more nutritious foods. Children need a balanced diet for normal growth and development. Although we do not seem to realise it, in our industrial countries it is not easy to find a child that is really healthy. Most children, especially those living in towns, are often listless and tired. They lack vitamins, minerals and other nutrients needed to fight and prevent stress.

Some children who are unable to express their stress in words will show it by their actions. They will suffer from anxiety and nightmares, become irritable, hyperactive, aggressive and afraid of sleeping alone; they may cower, run and bite, suffer from sleeping problems, or become accident-prone. Small children may even revert back to more immature behaviour, like sucking their thumbs, and fully toilet-trained children will suddenly start to wet their beds again. They may throw tantrums more frequently, or withdraw and become far too quiet.

The more severe the stress and the longer it lasts, the less control a child has over their reactions. The problem is that, nowadays, changes in our society and the lives of our children take place faster and faster, and the human organism cannot cope with so much stress. Parents should always try to prevent children being exposed to overwhelming stress, but this does not mean trying to keep them from experiencing normal, often healthy stresses. Children should learn that stress is a part of life and they should learn how to handle it. A sense of humour is extremely important. One should try to transform a negative, harmful experience so that it becomes a positive one that the child can overcome and learn from.

In coming to the end of this chapter, I would like to touch briefly on the tremendous results that people get from the Hara breathing exercise. It is quite remarkable what this exercise can do and I have already written extensively about it in my book *Stress and Nervous Disorders.* I think the reason why Professor Michael Gearin-Tosh put so much emphasis on this exercise in his book *The Living Proof* was because of the benefits he gained from this particular method of relaxation. He realised the extent to which stress influenced cancer – perhaps even triggering it. Being close to nature and undertaking Hara breathing has considerably lengthened his life. It is remarkable to think that when he was first diagnosed he was on the verge of giving up altogether.

It is also vital that the correct remedies are taken. Towards the end of last year, a lady came to me in a very distressed state. Like many people, she suffered additional health problems because of the dark days leading up to Christmas. I wrote down the Hara breathing exercise for her and asked her to try it. When she called to see me again last week, she told me about the tremendous improvement in her life since carrying out this technique. At her initial consultation, I also prescribed *Enhanced Nerve Factors* by Michael's, together with *Mood Essence, Concentration Essence* and *Relaxing Essence,* which are concocted from a combination of flower essences. Although that may seem like a lot of remedies to take, it was relatively little in comparison to the magnitude of her health problems. Within days, she told me she had become a new person. Being close to nature is a wonderful thing, and the flower essences that I created many years ago are now becoming even more important in this very stressful world in which we live, as they offer benefits in so many ways.

This chapter may seem quite complicated, but really stress management is so easy. As in the case of the last lady I mentioned, it might only be a matter of taking some simple remedies and carrying out some simple exercises to experience a new lease of life within a short space of time. It is therefore well worthwhile putting all your effort into improving your health and well-being.

CHAPTER EIGHT

How Much Sleep Do You Need?

One of the biggest concerns I have today is for those who cannot sleep. Never a day goes by in my practice without patients asking for my help in dealing with sleep deprivation – whether they suffer from insomnia, broken sleep or problems that have led to the disruption of their normal sleeping pattern. It is accepted that more than 10 million people in the UK suffer from sleep problems, and some have endured these for many years. Health and Safety Executive research has indicated that about half a million people experience work-related stress at a level they believe is making them ill. In 1995, the Department of Health estimated that 15.9 million prescriptions were written for sleeping pills and tranquillisers, at a cost of £22.3 million to the NHS. The pressures of life can very often lead to these problems.

Sleep remains a mystery, but what we do know is how sleep – or lack of it – affects us. What we do not know is how sleep works and why there is a need for it. Is there an ingredient in the blood which makes us sleep or is there some other cause? What causes our sleep to become disturbed? Although we know quite a bit about sleep, there is still much that we don't know. However, one thing is for sure, we cannot do without it. Sleep is essential so that the body can rest, completely relax and become energised again. Too little sleep can lead to headaches, lack of concentration, tiredness, irritability (and sometimes aggression) and also to a depletion of reserves.

I am often asked the question 'How much sleep do I really need?' The need for sleep is not the same for everyone, but I still advocate that the majority of people should have seven to eight hours' sleep a night. Some people say they only need four hours' sleep, whereas others may need eight. Our sleeping pattern changes as we get older. Babies and young children need a lot of sleep, while older people don't need as much. Strangely enough, those who say they can manage with little sleep are often deep sleepers. I greatly admired my old partner, Alfred Vogel, as he was usually in bed by nine o'clock, or ten o'clock at the latest. He worked on the principle that sleep during the hours before midnight was more valuable to the body than sleep during the hours after. He would then rise at four or five o'clock in the morning to work in his garden or to answer the hundreds of letters he received. I am often asked how I manage to work 90 hours a week. My answer is instantaneous – I have a God-given ability to sleep whenever and wherever I wish. If my body is exhausted, I can go off and have a sleep. After just half an hour of sleep, I feel fully energised.

If the quantity or quality of sleep is not as good as it should be, then positive action needs to be taken. All kinds of things can hinder people from sleeping soundly. It is necessary to make sure that if a problem is preventing you from sleeping, you do what you can to sort it out – but do not take it to bed with you.

In general, many people have forgotten how to live. The worst thing for an insomniac is to stay up late watching an exciting television programme. This results in the mind being overstimulated and overexcited. Cheese and crackers is often the snack that accompanies such a programme. Unfortunately, this will only exacerbate the situation, as cheese eaten shortly before bed adversely influences the sleep pattern.

It is necessary to look closely at your diet. Alcohol and spicy foods should be avoided, especially late at night. The last meal of the day should be taken approximately three to four hours before going to bed, as trying to sleep on a full stomach will cause additional problems. Instead of eating a large supper before bed, you should drink a cup of herbal tea, such as Melissa or Dutch herbal tea. Most people are aware that caffeine is a stimulant and is not conducive to sleep, so therefore avoid coffee, tea and hot chocolate drinks. I always warn people who come to our slimming clinic to avoid sugar. I have been encouraged by those who have managed to eliminate this from their diet, and even more so when some have reported that, after doing so, their sleeping patterns greatly improved.

One interesting factor I have observed in vegetarians is that they are usually good sleepers. I feel that eating meat can affect our nervous systems to the detriment of our sleeping patterns, and for that reason, I would like to say a little about meat here. In the past, meat was quite different from what it is now. Then, an animal which grazed on unpolluted grass or foraged in the wild provided much healthier meat than that which is available today. For a long time, meat was a luxury which most people could not afford. Later, it gradually became cheaper, and now almost everyone can afford it. Today, meat has been given the place of honour, while vegetables and other foods do not seem to be quite so important any more for most people who live in the industrial countries.

There are millions of people in the world who do not eat meat and are nevertheless healthy. Eating is something very personal, and eating meat is no exception. Although the meat we eat today is certainly not one of our healthiest foods, there are people who obviously need the satisfaction which they derive from eating it. It seems to give them a pleasure one could call addictive. If these people do not eat meat more than twice a week, it probably will not harm them – the pleasure they find in eating will counterbalance the possible negative effects meat may have on their health. Here, 'mind over matter' is very important.

Many religions do not permit the consumption of pork. This is not only for religious reasons but also for reasons of health. Pork contains much fat and provides ideal living conditions for germs and viruses. It can therefore cause all kinds of diseases. Pork and pork products are definitely not healthy foods.

After you have had your dinner, instead of sitting in front of the television all evening, it would be much healthier to take a short walk – perhaps with the dog – or a short cycle ride, so that you feel totally relaxed before going to bed. Also ensure that your bed is comfortable and that your bedroom is at the right temperature – neither too hot nor too cold. It is a good idea to open the window slightly, allowing fresh air to circulate.

If you can't sleep, then try playing some soft background music or perhaps try some light reading, preferably something humorous. An elderly patient once told me she could not sleep at all. I recommended she watch *Dad's Army* before going to bed. Whenever she sees me now, she tells me that she has the entire collection of *Dad's Army* tapes because watching that does the trick for her!

Some people who find it difficult to get to sleep resort to counting sheep, but the Hara breathing exercises that I advocate in my book *Stress and Nervous Disorders* are very helpful. A gentle massage can also be extremely beneficial. You could relax by unwinding in a warm bath to which a few drops of lavender oil have been added, or even trying some reflexology.

Sleep is not difficult. It is the most natural thing in the world and there is no substitute for it. However, it is sometimes necessary to 'learn' how to sleep. So, before going to bed, try some gentle exercise, switch off your mind with some pleasant thoughts, leave your worries to one side and trust your own body. It will work for you as long as you give it a chance. After a good night's sleep, you will waken up in the morning feeling refreshed, healthy and ready to face another day.

Please do not rely on drugs, as they will make you feel like a zombie and will not cure the problem. A good alternative would be some natural remedies which are not addictive or habit-forming. A wonderful way to relax and aid restful sleep is to use Alfred Vogel's *St John's Wort Oil* or to sprinkle a few drops of lavender, rosemary or geranium oil on your pillowslip.

As everyone knows, the digestive system slows down at night, and it would therefore be a good idea to drink a cup of Melissa herbal tea, as already mentioned, or some camomile tea. If these do not have the desired effect, then try some herbs, such as *A. Vogel Valerian-Hops Complex* (20 to 30 drops to be taken half an hour before going to bed), which have a calming and sedating effect. In dealing with a stressful situation, I find *Nux vomica* to be a marvellous remedy, and taking two *Calm Repose* tablets from Abbots of Leigh can often work wonders.

The lymphatic system, which only works while we are asleep, does a superb job in cleansing our blood. If there is too much waste material in our lymph glands, we can experience problems. Very often, the tired people who come along to my clinics are suffering from this. Lymph swellings are full of toxic materials, resulting in the system being unable to function properly. This is often the case with ME patients, especially those who have suffered glandular fever.

During sleep, the lymphatic system is cleansed. If one cannot sleep, it is wise to take a natural remedy such as *Valerian-Hops Complex,* as mentioned earlier. Alternatively, it would be beneficial to take a very good antioxidant preparation, such as *Doctor's Choice Antioxidant* or Michael's *Antioxidant,* to help clear the lymphatic system. It is imperative that you ensure your lymphatic system is functioning to its maximum ability. If it isn't, you should consult a qualified and experienced doctor or practitioner for guidance. I have seen numerous illnesses and diseases develop from a congested lymphatic system.

Being unable to sleep undoubtedly causes tremendous problems. You can lie awake for hours, tossing and turning. In the middle of the night, worries appear to be of insurmountable magnitude. The problems that you have experienced during the day or those that lie ahead can really destroy your body. It is therefore vital that you try to recognise any anxieties before they escalate, and eliminate them as best you can. Remember that going to bed on a full stomach will only add to your problems, and if you follow my advice, taking the remedies I have mentioned, then you will hopefully start to regard sleep as a friend. It is still true that the hours spent asleep before midnight are worth double those after midnight. Don't overtax your brain. Try to improve your ability to relax and repeat inwardly, 'I want to relax, I want to relax.' Make sure that you put your mind totally at ease before going to bed so that you can enjoy a relaxed and peaceful night's sleep.

CHAPTER NINE

How to Enjoy Gentle Exercise

In this day and age when society has changed so much – and often for the worse – it is important that everyone undertakes some form of exercise. Most of us are guilty of sitting – and standing – too much and not doing the correct exercises that are needed for the human body. In contrast, our ancestors probably did too much exercise and work, but nowadays we don't use our body, arms, legs or even our spine the way we should. For that reason, embarking upon some method of exercise can do nothing but benefit us all.

I repeatedly advise patients who are suffering from stiffness or pain in their back and neck to choose exercises that are pertinent to their particular complaint. Walking, swimming and cycling are excellent for good mobility. It is equally important – or even more so – for those suffering from a degenerative disease, who have restricted movement and pain and discomfort, to carry out some gentle, simple exercises that do not overtax the body.

It is vital that serious thought is given to the exercises that are most appropriate for you before engaging in ones which may ultimately prove to be totally unsuitable. For example, when a patient suffering from back and neck problems enthusiastically tells me how aerobic exercises are good for them, I have to contradict them by saying that they are not suitable for their particular problem and that they would achieve more benefits from trying an alternative method.

We are currently spoiled for choice by the wide range of exercises available to suit all our requirements – from simple exercises to the Alexander technique, Pilates or the Caesar technique. This chapter is intended to make you aware of the more straightforward exercises that can be carried out in a simple manner to improve health and vitality, yet achieve great results.

Relaxing exercises are not only vital for our bones and muscles, but also for our spine. Osteoporosis has become a huge problem and is often made worse by lack of exercise. It is essential that we give careful thought to whichever part of our body needs attention. Bone marrow, cartilage, muscle, vertebrae and tissues all have to function well, and pain can often be the result of insufficient exercise.

If possible, try and have a look at the exercises I have described in some of my books – especially those in *Neck and Back Problems* and the hydrotherapy exercises mentioned in *Water: Healer or Poison?*

When we experience pain in the spine, we need to be aware that this can be attributed to long hours spent in front of a computer. Even just sitting for long periods can lead to many problems. When the back suddenly 'goes', as my patients often say, this can be as a result of improper lifting. When lifting objects, it is imperative that you bend your knees, not your back. Carrying out easy exercises on a regular basis can protect the back, which is a much more responsible approach than trying to cure the problem once the pain has taken hold. Back problems usually involve muscles and ligaments, and often nerve inflammation.

Excessive or inappropriate exercising can easily damage the back. Be careful when involving yourself in activities that may be too much for you. It is for this reason that I advise you to be choosy in what exercise you decide to tackle. A lot of damage can be done by unknowingly moving incorrectly. In a nutshell, the main thing is to keep your spine as straight as possible. Good posture is extremely important. Don't overload yourself with heavy bags, and take notice when your neck or back gives a twinge, as this is indicative of something being wrong.

Patients often tell me that they have had a wonderful evening out, but that they had to sit too long either in the same position or beside an open window, resulting in a sore back or neck. A good remedy for this is to have a hot bath to which some bicarbonate of soda has been added when you get home. Also try this simple exercise as a means of relieving tension in the neck: move your head in a circular motion clockwise; do this five times and then repeat the same action again, but this time in an anticlockwise direction.

A hot bicarbonate of soda bath will also relieve overworked or overstretched muscles following sporting activities. It is a simple task to protect muscles from becoming painful. It is vital to warm up properly before starting an exercise routine and to use *Arnica Gel* if your muscles are sore, then you won't need to worry about having a constant pain that could take ages to move.

A visit to a reputable practitioner in manual therapy or a good masseur can be extremely helpful. They will also be able to talk you through beneficial ways in which to relax by using the most appropriate exercises for your particular problem.

General body massage is recognised as an ideal means of keeping the body in a healthy condition. Massage offers an invaluable aid in the treatment of bodily ills and is of tremendous help in cases of obesity, diabetes and other conditions. Poor circulation and other conditions which put pressure on the heart will also be helped greatly by general massage. In these cases, massage, by increasing the circulation, relieves the heart and other organs of their burden. It has to be realised that many important organs and tissues of the body which cannot be directly reached by massage are nevertheless stimulated indirectly through the nervous system, and also by improving the circulation, respiration and elimination. I also advocate Hara breathing or very deep breathing exercises as another way of invigorating and promoting good circulation.

Hydrotherapy is a wonderful way to exercise. Not only swimming but, as explained in my book *Water: Healer or Poison?*, hydrotherapy treatments and exercises will give the most amazing results and are a gentle way to keep fit.

Remedial exercises may be defined as the scientific application of bodily movements designed to maintain or restore normal muscle and joint function. Unlike in massage, there has been no attempt to give names to the various movements in remedial exercises. However, the movements have been arranged to follow a definite sequence or order of many positions. These remedial exercises can be done by oneself or with a therapist. Joint movements through exercises are important. It is therefore not a waste of money to see a good remedial therapist who will help with these gentle exercises to relax the whole body.

Practitioners can be of tremendous help but, for those who find this course of action outwith their budget, there is a lot one can do by carrying out simple procedures to aid rest and relaxation when problems surface. So, if you have a sore back, you could try these simple methods at home before consulting a therapist. Place two large pillows on the floor, lie face down with the pillows under your stomach and breathe deeply in through the nose and out through the mouth. You could also try lying on a bed on your right side, then placing one pillow between the knees and drawing the knees up towards the chest. These are excellent ways of relieving pain.

Our body can be likened to the battery of a car. The right side is positive and the left side is negative, and if these are balanced with the proper exercises, then we will see how much can be done. Gravity is most important. If Isaac Newton had known what can be achieved with the laws of gravity and how the centre of gravity is important to balance left and right, he would have been amazed! This is what acupuncture is all about.

The energies which are generally inaccessible to the five senses, such as the meridian flow, chakras and auras, are often guided by intuition. We see this in the proper practice of shiatsu. This Japanese healing art depends on an interactive balance between the energy of the practitioner and that of the patient. It allows the patient to get in touch with their own healing powers. This is one of the reasons why I am keen to promote Hara breathing – these exercises enable the patient to maintain the energy balance achieved in shiatsu sessions.

I would reiterate that, in today's society, exercise is more necessary than ever, and it is up to us which methods we decide upon. Perhaps you might choose horse riding, basketball, rowing, tennis, badminton or golf, but whatever you settle on, you must look at the balance in your exercise regime. I have seen a lot of famous golfers in my life – even some world champions – with irreparable back damage, and I have stressed over and over again that the balance of energy is important. Most golfers put enormous pressure on only one side of their body, but it is vital to use all our bones and muscles in order to balance our energy. Because of this, I advise them to try swimming or any other form of exercise that will use both sides of the body equally. It is a similar situation with footballers. I have had the privilege of treating many famous footballers in my life. However, I have had to educate many in the ways of balancing the body to counteract the strain they put on themselves.

I like the idea of the barefoot practitioners using the reflexes in their feet, and the thought of carrying out exercises on the dewy grass early in the morning. In some cases, this might prove difficult, but it would make a most refreshing start to the day for many town dwellers who are confined to their rooms and offices to experience this at the start of their day.

In my book *Body Energy*, I detailed many hand movements which show what can be done using your own hands to help to balance the body's own energy. Small movements using gentle pressure, which are also used in cranial osteopathy, can offer relief to the whole body. It is quite interesting to see how the body appreciates this help.

I give examples of some of these hand positions over the following pages. If practised regularly, this kind of exercise will help the individual to rebalance specific energy problems and will also promote a general improvement in mind–body balance. Depending on the individual, the effectiveness of some positions may diminish after repeated use, whereas others will be found beneficial even after they have been used many times. If you wish to find out more about these exercises, I would recommend consulting an energy specialist, such as a reiki practitioner, who will be able to advise you on which positions would be of most benefit to you.

The hand positions illustrated are not always symmetrical; one hand may be held in a different manner to the other. Thus, when trying a particular position, you may feel more comfortable with left and right hands reversed. In this case, the position which you find more comfortable should always be used.

The vast majority of these hand positions will not draw undue attention to the user and certain ones will be of great benefit when used in the presence of others, particularly in the presence of persons who are using energy to the detriment of others around them.

Some of the positions, however, will provide the most benefit in rebalancing or meditation when practised while alone, and a number of these will be beneficial even when practised while the user is sleeping. The use of a stocking or other device may be required to hold the hands in the desired position, thus dispensing with the need for the conscious mind to concentrate on holding the position.

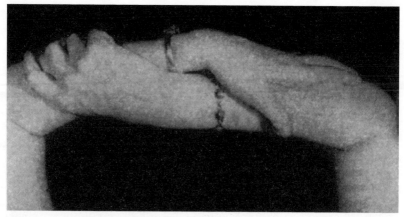

Own true self (1)

This position is used to bring the sense of action to rest. It is useful for isolating oneself in the presence of moderate energy. Each forearm is grasped by the opposite hand. The ankles may also be crossed at the same time.

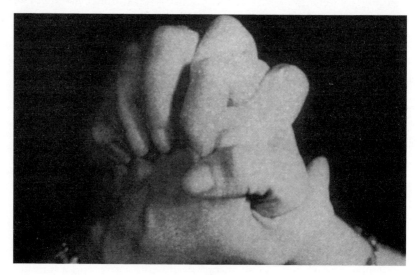

Own true self (2)

This is used to induce quiet perception. The hands are clasped, with the fingers and thumbs externally intertwined.

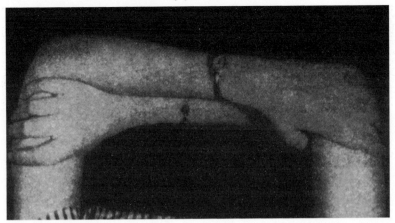

Own true self (3)

Use this position to isolate oneself in the presence of heavy and disturbing energy. Each upper arm is grasped by the opposite hand.

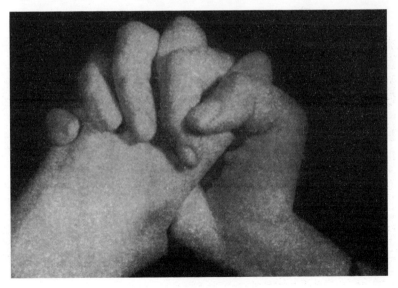

Own true self (4)

This position is used to balance yin and yang in the body. The fingers and thumbs are externally intertwined, with the free thumb placed under the wrist of the other hand.

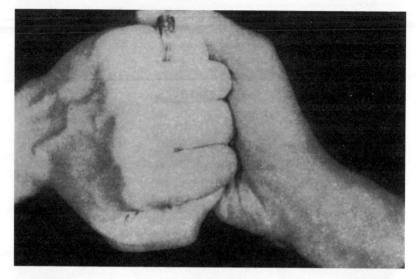

Keying things out

This position helps to calm a person down. It also has a neutralising effect on various parts of the body, such as the stomach and eyes. The fingers of each hand are hooked and firmly engage each other. Each thumb lies along the little finger of the opposite hand.

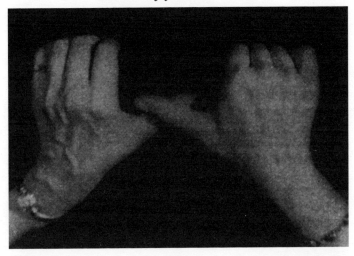

Step 1

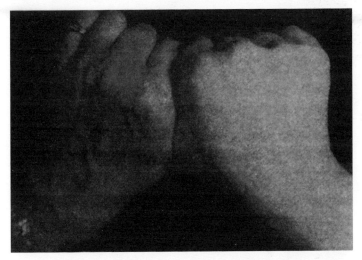

Step 2

This position is used to send energy quickly and automatically to where it is needed at any point in the body. It can be used for breaking up congestions. The thumb of each hand is grasped between the fingers and palm of the opposite hand. The position is easily entered by first crossing the thumbs (Step 1) and sliding the hands together before closing the fingers (Step 2).

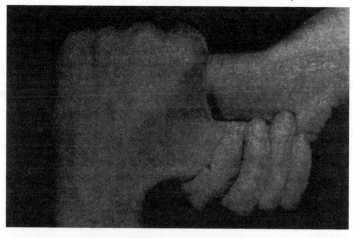

Getting in the positive

Use this position to correct negative attitudes. This is the same position as the previous one, except that the hands are rotated so that one wrist is up and the other wrist is down.

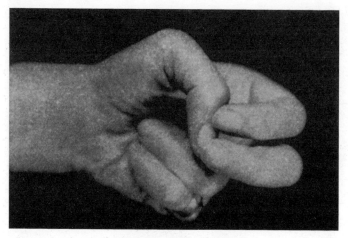

Activating without energy

This position helps to keep the mind alert in the absence of energy and is used when the hands cannot be brought together. The ring and little fingers are held against the palm and the tips of the forefinger and middle finger are placed above the first joint of the thumb.

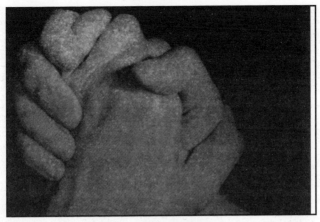

Foreground awareness

This position promotes the inner self and also serves to de-energise. With the fingers held together, the palms are placed to face each other at right angles and then the fingers and thumbs are wrapped around the opposite hand.

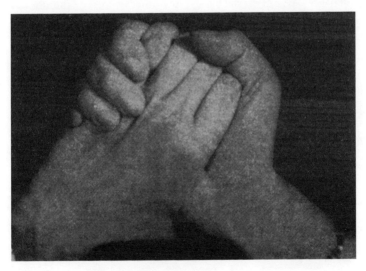

Background awareness

This is used to pull oneself together and protect from energy domination by another person. It is the same as the previous clasp except that the free thumb is placed behind the opposite wrist.

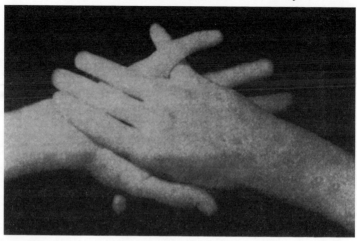

Without will-power

This position helps to release emotions that have been withheld. The palm of one hand is placed on the back of the other hand. The thumbs and little fingers are interlocked.

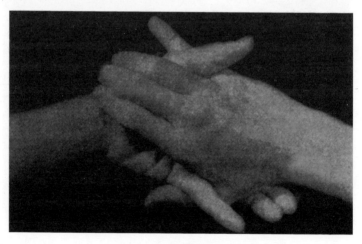

As of now

This position has an immediate impact on the senses and aids rebalancing. The hands are held flat and placed palm to palm. The thumb of each hand is interlocked with the little finger of the opposite hand.

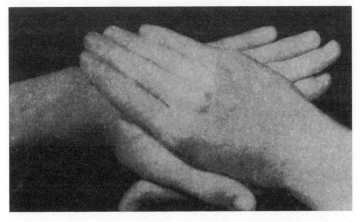

Neutralising

This position promotes a calm mind and aids in meditation. It also neutralises unbalanced body conditions when the hands are held in this way and placed over a deficient body part, such as a tense stomach. One hand is held flat and placed on the back of the other and the thumbs are interlocked.

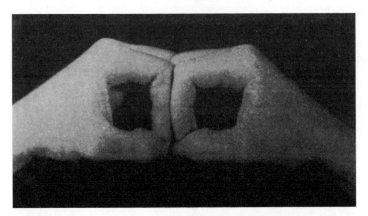

Quiet hands (1)

This position is used to quieten the forebrain. The fingertips are placed in line and bent over to make a circle, with each thumb tip touching the tip of the forefinger. The backs of the knuckles of all the fingers are brought together.

225

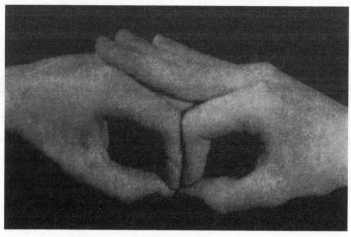

Quiet hands (2)

This quietens the midbrain. A circle is made with each thumb and forefinger, with the three remaining fingers of each hand remaining extended and together. The extended fingers of one hand are placed on top of those of the other hand.

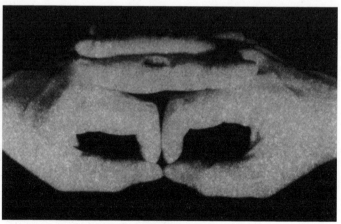

Quiet hands (3)

This quietens the hindbrain. This is the same as the previous position, except that the extended fingers are externally intertwined, or interlaced.

226

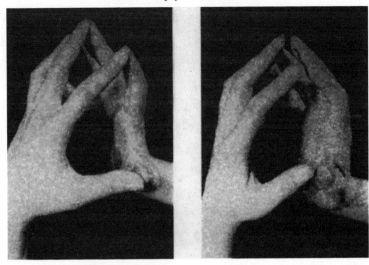

Talking without energy

This position improves the flow of energy from one person to another. It also keeps the mind on business rather than personalities. With the fingers spread apart, a cup is made out of each hand. The corresponding fingertips are brought together and then separated again by about half an inch. Do this once every 1–2 seconds, or even less often if that seems more comfortable.

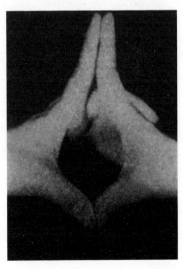

With this position, flows are generated which help the self and others in the vicinity to be rebalanced through foreground awareness. The little fingers, ring fingers and middle fingers are externally interlaced. The forefingers and thumbs are extended in opposite directions, with the tips of the thumbs and the tips of the fingers placed together.

Creating positive energy (1)

227

This time, flows are generated which help the self and others in the vicinity to be rebalanced through background awareness. This position also triggers the flow of key-ins which have become stuck in the background awareness. The ring fingers, middle fingers and forefingers are externally interlaced. The tips of the little fingers and the tips of the thumbs are brought together.

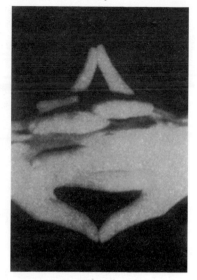

Creating positive energy (2)

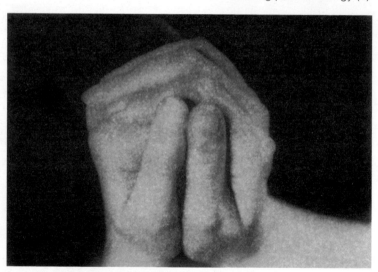

Rebalancing with visualisation wide open

The closed fist of one hand is covered with the other hand and the two thumbs are held alongside each other.

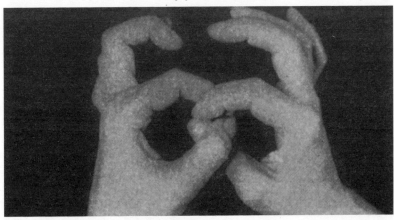

Step 1

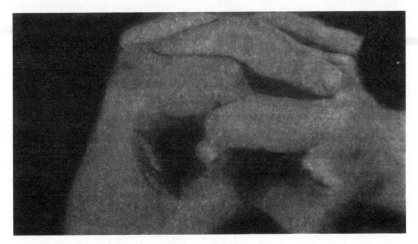

Step 2

Rebalancing natural emotions

This position encourages energies to flow from the body to the mind. A pair of interlocked chain links is made with the thumbs and forefingers (Step 1). The remaining three fingers of each hand are then interlaced in such a way that the middle finger and ring finger of the lower hand come between the middle finger and ring finger of the upper hand. The point where the chain links cross is maintained at the forefinger and thumb tips; all four of these should be in contact with one another (Step 2).

229

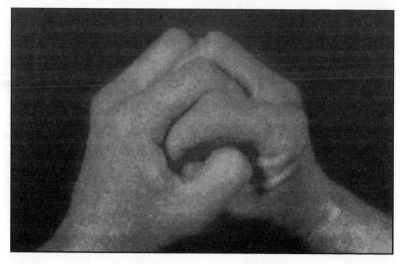

Coordinating the two halves of the brain

All fingers and thumbs are internally interlaced.

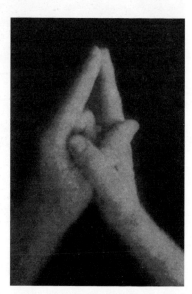

The little fingers, ring fingers and middle fingers are internally interlaced. The forefingers are extended and made to touch each other at the tips. The thumbs are crossed.

Coordinating the neck

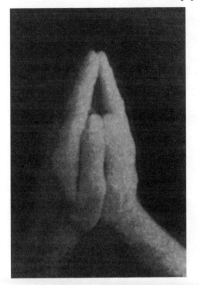

The little fingers, ring fingers and middle fingers are internally interlaced. The forefingers and thumbs are extended. The thumbs are held alongside each other and the forefingers touch each other at the tips.

Coordinating the backbone

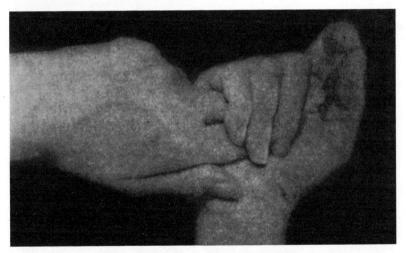

Sharpening the mind for business activity

The thumb, forefinger and middle finger of the first hand are placed in the palm of the second hand and grasped by the little finger, ring finger and middle finger of the second hand. A circle is made by bringing together the tips of the forefinger and thumb of the second hand. The little finger and ring finger of the first hand are closed against the palm of that hand.

231

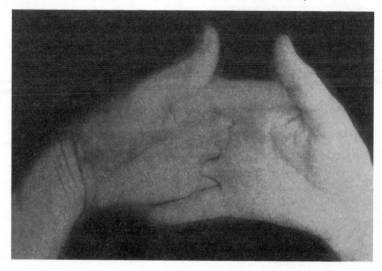

Inducing relaxation

The fingers, but not the thumbs, are externally interlaced. The combined palms are then placed over the body part that requires to be relaxed, for example the eyes, forehead or jaw.

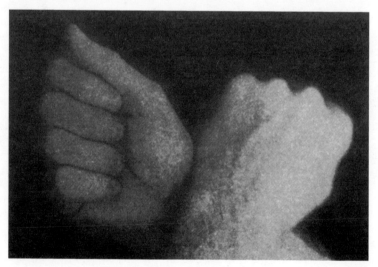

Rebalancing will-power

Each hand is made into a fist and the two wrists are crossed at right angles so as to touch each other on the inside.

MAGNETISM

I cannot help thinking what a tremendous future there is in the reflex techniques that I use in electromagnetic stimulation. This is a relaxing exercise technique which has great potential, and when Dr Len Allan and I worked together on this in the 1970s, we discovered how much benefit there was in giving magnetic treatments. Magnetism can be a powerful healing force, and for that reason I'd like to go into the subject in more detail here.

Magnetic forces were used in healing as early as 1772, when Franz Anton Mesmer, an Austrian physician, began to investigate the curative powers of the magnet and formed the opinion that there exists a power similar to magnetism that exercises an extraordinary influence on the human body. After Mesmer's theories fell into disrepute, magnetism was for a long time ignored by modern medicine. This was probably due to the impossibility in the past of measuring these forces and the subsequent unpredictability of the results. Later, the subject was elevated from the domain of charlatanism to that of scientific research.

The movement of an external magnetic force interacting with the body's inner electrical field will generate a weak current, but only when this current reaches a certain intensity will results be observed.

In the eighteenth century, the artificial magnets made by Father Hall, the celebrated astronomer of Vienna, were used in the form of magnetic armatures and helped to relieve spasms, convulsions and paralyses.

In France, Abbot Lenoble succeeded in making the strongest artificial magnets yet created, and, in 1771, he began testing their therapeutic applications. He applied certain pieces, such as magnetic bracelets and crosses, to the wrist, chest and so on, and observed benefits to the subjects. In 1777, he reported his findings to the Royal Society of Medicine and invited them to verify them. The Royal

Society entrusted two of their members, Andry and Thouret, with the repetition of his experiments.

They conducted 48 tests, the cases observed including toothache, nervous pains in the head and loins, rheumatic pains, facial neuralgia, tic douloureux, stomach spasms, spasmodic hiccups, palpitations, different kinds of tremor, convulsions and epilepsy. Among the effects observed, a large number occurred a short time after the application of the magnet. In some cases, sharp neuralgic pains in the face were soothed by the contact of the magnet. Spasmodic and convulsive symptoms disappeared rapidly after the application of the magnet; a nervous cough was instantly soothed and did not reappear. In one case, convulsive movements of the arm and contracture ceased or were notably diminished in the course of the day. Rheumatic pains were soothed, and in cases where they returned after the removal of the magnet, they disappeared upon replacing it. In others, similar pains, calmed by the action of the magnet, appeared again in different parts of the body. They were dissipated by the local application of the pole of a magnet. In cases of toothache, the application of the magnet was sometimes followed by prompt and obvious relief. At times, when a magnet did not soothe pains or other symptoms, against which it had been effective in other patients, relief was gained by prolonging the application or by using a stronger magnet.

Following Andry and Thouret, several other observers, among whom may be mentioned Marcellin, Halle, Laennec, Albert, Cayol, Chomel, Recamier and Alexander Lebreton, tested the truth of the majority of these observations.

Armand Trousseau says in the *Dictionnaire de Médecine,* published in 1833:

> As for us, who have sometimes made use of the magnet, we can state that this therapeutic agent exercises an influence over

other parts with which it comes into contact, an influence which it is impossible to refer to the patient's imagination. I have seen neuralgic pains modified, attacks of nervous dysnopea [shortness of breath] checked, etc. Laennec is gratified with the effects of the magnet in the treatment of angina pectoris. I have been able to gather two facts myself which prove that, if the magnet does not cure disease, it can at least moderate its intensity. Incontestable cures have been performed in cases of rheumatism, temporarily it is true, but in support of this we can cite the history of a French marshal whose rheumatic pains could only be relieved by the use of magnetic armatures. It is not claimed that the application of a magnet to a painful area will relieve the pain in every case, so many factors being involved in its production.

Instead of the patient having to resort to taking a drug to alleviate their discomfort, magnet therapy should be tried. Its use certainly cannot do any harm – something which cannot be said of any drug.

In the treatment of the spine, the prongs of the magnet should be placed astride the upper spine and then gently and slowly drawn downwards to the end of the spinal column, twenty times or so, each stroke to take one minute to complete.

Unknown effects can be produced in the body and the body may have the ability to respond to these forces. Based on this hypothesis, we conducted clinical experiments at my clinic at Auchenkyle with various lengths, sizes and types of magnets and developed two methods of magnetic interaction. The first uses a wide magnetic field of 500 gauss or more, which produces local analgesia. The second method employs a mild magnetic force which, when applied continuously to a certain point, will produce a meridian effect, sending energy all over the body.

For example, if a magnetic force of 1,000 gauss or more is applied to local pain areas, a remarkable painkilling effect (similar to that of acupuncture) is observed immediately after treatment.

Magnetic Energy Flow

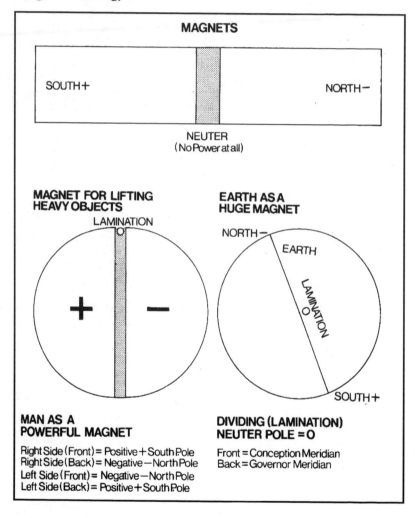

The diagram above shows the reason for the energy flow at the ends of a magnet. In reality, there are three poles to all magnets – the positive,

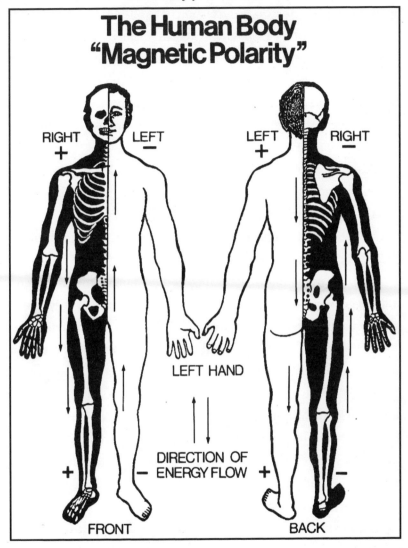

The Human Body "Magnetic Polarity"

RIGHT +   LEFT −   LEFT +   RIGHT −

LEFT HAND

DIRECTION OF ENERGY FLOW

+ −   + −

FRONT   BACK

The flow of magnetic energy in the human body

negative and neuter. This is the main reason for the polar intensity of attraction and repulsion at its ends. Have a look at the illustration, which shows a positive (south) pole and also a negative (north) pole. Somewhere along its length, towards its centre, is a neutral zone or neuter pole, where there is no attraction or repulsion. It is at this point that both polar energies flow and return to their respective poles. Observe the huge magnets used in industry to lift heavy items – these are usually composed of two magnets: the north pole of one and the south pole of the other, separated by a lamination which acts like the neutral zone of a magnet. This is what gives the industrial magnet its tremendous power for lifting.

Taking it a step further, even this earth of ours has its lamination, or neutral zone, the north–south line, and also the division of the equator, two hemispheres divided as is the industrial magnet.

The human body is no exception to the law, as the right side of the body is the positive (south) pole and the negative (north) pole is the left side. Its lamination is, according to the Chinese, the conception and the governor meridians. It is true of all magnets that they have a triune quality – they are positive, negative and neutral at once. It is this neutral zone, in all matter and magnets, that enhances the polar power of attraction and repulsion in all magnets.

The World of Magnetism

The earth has its own magnetism or magnetic force, which also involves gravity. This force is duplicated in the human body, and we can learn how to use it. God and nature have given man, and earth, this magnetic force from the very beginning of the world. The earth's own magnetism, and what man has researched and devised, can and does affect every living system on the face of this earth, the space above the earth and even to the very core of the earth. It is now beginning to be known that it affects all biological systems, even down to micro-organisms in all matter.

It is now known that we, from the first day of our existence, and animals, seeds and plants from the first day of theirs, are born into the earth's existing magnetic field. Any changes in this energy field can and do affect the health and welfare of all living systems.

Magnetism is a force rather than an energy and the idea is to get this force to emanate away from the magnet and not back on itself. The only way people who are working with this energy can do anything with magnetism is to attract the force through the tissue by placing the tissue to be treated between two opposite poles.

Bio-Electromagnetic Reflexes

There is a law of physics in electromagnetics which states that any wire carrying a current produces a magnetic field. Since this law is always constant, any nerve carrying impulses produces a magnetic field. The type of impulse and the consistency and duration of the impulse determines what type of magnetic field is created – south pole (positive) or north pole (negative).

Under normal conditions, our body is automatically controlled by our brain. Only when there is a disturbance do the nerves start sending messages, or impulses, to the brain for it to correct the problem, either with more blood to heal, cells to replace others, plasma for repair, spasms for protection, etc. Usually, electrical impulses, or energy, start to create a magnetic field, measurable through a like polarity distortion factor (especially in the legs). Prolonged and continued impulses create one type of field, and continued unanswered impulses create another type of field.

The use of a unipolar magnet or modified phased magnet unit can reveal the visceral somatic reflexes which pass through the spinal centres connected with an organ or part. These are the autonomic connections between the tissues and the central nervous system. One can, with training and some medical knowledge, see these visceral somatic reflexes, which lead to a new understanding of the problems and the causes of the conditions seen in the average patient visiting the office.

Any *negative* reading means the organ or part is irritated, over-energised, hypertonic and almost always in a state of tension in muscle areas. It is also likely to be a painful spot.

Any *positive* reading means the part is really toneless, paralysed and not functioning properly or normally. It is devitalised and weak, and stretched by the opposing stronger muscles. It is usually painful from overstretching and weakness. The specific interpretation of the diagnosis is made through the magnetic fields and their locations, and can always be checked at the autonomic connections with the spinal column.

The types of diseases and conditions found in most patients are almost always the result of malfunctions of the basic organs involved, these being the liver, kidneys, intestines and bowels, and the other organs and endocrines to a much lesser degree. From the main organs stem all of the toxic factors which create secondary pathology, such as head and chest conditions, skin conditions, painful muscles and nerves, bad shoulders, neck and arms, back, hip and leg conditions. Rarely is a strain or spasm primary – it is usually the result of an underlying pathology.

I was basically very sceptical about the magnetic bracelets that are widely recommended until I started to research them a bit more. Magnetic forces are much stronger than one can ever imagine, and I find that whatever is used to balance energy in this day and age, magnetic forces have an important part to play. Sometimes these simple methods, although unconventional, will help, and as long as they improve our health and increase our vitality, then they have a great purpose.

CHAPTER TEN

The Best of Sexual Health

One of the reasons I decided to include a chapter in this book on the subject of sexual health was a visit from a female patient. This particular lady sat across from me one morning telling me how overjoyed she was that not only had I saved her marriage but that her life had become much more enjoyable. When she first came to see me, she was in tears as she told me of her problem, which was not only painful and unpleasant but also totally restricted her sexual activities. She had herpes zoster. This is a viral condition which can never actually be cleared but, fortunately, can be kept under control. She told me that she had developed an inferiority complex as a result of this and that she found it distressing. She didn't know how she had contracted it, but the preceding few years had been a nightmare as she felt it all very embarrassing. She told me that she was a chef in a top hotel but since she had contracted this virus she felt that her job had become too taxing. As she had no alternative but to continue working, her life had become extremely difficult.

After we discussed her diet, I told her to make some necessary changes to make it much healthier. I then advised her to carry out a complete detoxification programme, which she was keen to do, and she chose Vogel's *Detox Box.* Following that, I prescribed an effective blood detoxification treatment from Michael's and, subsequently, *ViraPlex* from Enzymatic (one tablet twice a day), a large dose of *Echinaforce,* and *R68,* which is a homoeopathic remedy from Dr Reckeweg, at a dosage of fifteen drops twice daily. Within a few weeks, the condition had cleared, her life had improved dramatically and her intimate relationship with her husband had been restored to its former state. She has since written to me a few times about this nasty virus, concerned that it could return.

Many people have consulted me regarding this problem, which is more widespread than one thinks. However, if my advice is followed to the letter, it can usually be kept under control. It would be dishonest to say that herpes simplex or herpes zoster, both viral conditions, can be cleared completely. Sometimes it may be necessary to repeat the aforementioned treatment. Because of the very unpleasant and drastic way that this virus attacks the body, it can put relationships under enormous strain. However, this is only one of the many conditions that can lead to difficulties in a relationship.

The other day, a middle-aged lady consulted me. She told me that her life was being ruined by a nasty infection called thrush, which had persisted for a long time. Thrush, also called candidiasis, is a common fungal condition which causes itching and/or soreness around the entrance of the vagina, making sexual intercourse very uncomfortable. There may also be a thick, whitish discharge. It is more common in women who are diabetic, who are (or have been) on antibiotics and who are on the contraceptive pill. The increased hormone level causes changes in the vaginal environment that make it perfect for fungal growth. It can be sexually transmitted and men can be carriers, although often they do not show any symptoms. This situation can lead to difficulties in an otherwise close relationship.

Although it is something which would usually be completely against my principles, I have to advise people with thrush to avoid fresh vegetables and fresh fruit. As the chlorophyll in fresh vegetables and fruits often lengthens the duration of the infection, it is advisable to eat cooked, steamed or dried vegetables and fruit in this instance. This can often clear the condition up quickly. There are also some herbal remedies which offer tremendous help in treating thrush, such as *Solidago Complex* (golden rod) and *Spilanthes*. As with any candida problem, *Yeast Balance* from Enzymatic is an effective remedy. Over the years, the problems that I have been able to conquer for people with these conditions have been countless, and this is one of the reasons I decided to write about it in this book. It is all part of good health and vitality.

I have also treated hundreds of people with spinal problems during my lifetime, and when there is a spinal condition such as a slipped disc (which is the common name for a prolapse in the vertebral disc), this can cause great difficulty in performing any sexual act. It is therefore important when such a problem is present, whether it be a lumbar, cervical or spondylitical condition, that the advice given by the doctor is taken. You must also ensure that no pressure is put on the area in question.

A problem that causes a lot of frustration is when there is pain during intercourse. This can have various possible causes, such as chronic prostatic infection, scars in the urethra, overtight foreskin, allergy of the penis or inflammation in either partner. Fortunately, these can be easily solved with some simple homoeopathic remedies, although if you have any problem that might lead to an infection, or if there already is any infection either of the vagina or the penis, this should be reported to your doctor immediately, especially as the

243

cause could be a venereal disease that might lead to much more serious problems unless treated with the appropriate medication.

One day, a young man arrived on the doorstep of one of my clinics. I had seen him a few months previously and was worried about him because I felt that an underlying problem was definitely making him suicidal. I eventually managed to persuade him to see his doctor. Luckily, the doctor diagnosed his condition and quickly got his problem cleared with the use of some strong antibiotics. He had contracted gonorrhoea. He was extremely worried about the situation but felt too embarrassed to confide in anyone about it, even his own doctor. He thought that if he came to me, I could give him something that would help. Unfortunately, I realised this would not be the case and that strong action would have to be taken. As he was grateful for my advice, he had now returned to thank me for saving his life. If left untreated, gonorrhoea can cause additional problems and may ultimately lead to kidney failure. It is one of the most common infectious bacterial diseases and is most frequently transmitted during sexual intercourse. It is therefore imperative that your partner is told. If you develop any symptoms, such as painful urination or discharge from the penis or vagina, you should see your doctor without delay.

Another man comes to my mind who was also suicidal, because his relationship was suffering greatly as a result of his problem with premature ejaculation. This is a common complaint from which many men suffer and which can lead to sexual dissatisfaction on the part of either or both partners and discord in a relationship. He had not sought help for this; instead he and his partner had tried to deal with the problem themselves. It is important that such difficulties are discussed in a relationship. Because this complaint is often psychological, men must not fear to ask for help from either their doctor or a sex therapist. Women have an important role to play in helping their partners overcome their possible feelings of guilt or lowered self-esteem by offering them reassurance. There are several issues which can lead to premature ejaculation – it can be the fear of making a woman pregnant, worry or some other psychological or physical cause. Steps can be taken to eliminate embarrassment or feelings of inadequacy. This particular man was greatly helped by taking excellent remedies called *Stress-End* and *A. Vogel Avena Sativa* from Bioforce. He managed to solve his problem completely and was able to enjoy a fulfilling sexual relationship again.

Another problem that I often come across is a urinary or bladder condition. This is a complaint suffered by both men and women for which there is a wide range of possible diagnoses. It could be an infection, a short urethra (which allows germs to multiply more easily), inflammation, a nasty bladder diverticulum or a problem of bladder capacity. Whatever the reason, this must be dealt with in order to maintain or improve sexual health. It will be helpful to carry out pelvic-floor exercises and to use a few remedies to eliminate the continual need to urinate, such as *Uva-ursi Complex* or *Golden Rod.* It may also be valuable to ask for guidance in some simple exercises from a physiotherapist.

Bladder inflammation, usually known as cystitis, is one of the most widespread infections. When the lining of the bladder becomes irritated and inflamed, there can even be blood present in the urine. Cystitis is often considered to be a minor illness, but it can actually lead to tremendous problems. The symptoms of cystitis are a burning, stinging or aching pain when you pass urine; a need to pass water more frequently, but often only a small amount each time; and cloudy urine. It can lead to more serious problems such as bladder weakness or incontinence. Although this can be an embarrassing situation in a relationship, it can easily be cleared up. If there is any blood in the urine, always seek medical advice. Plenty of water, Dutch herbal tea or *Golden Rod* tea are all beneficial in the treatment of bladder infections.

Other conditions such as period problems, heavy periods, vaginal discharge, premenstrual syndrome, osteoporosis, cervical erosions, endometriosis, fibroids, pelvic inflammatory disease, prolapse, menopausal symptoms and heart disease can all inhibit a healthy sex life. These particular problems can be addressed by a doctor or specialist, or, alternatively, by a naturopath, who has a variety of remedies at his disposal to give additional help.

The body is really a wonderful thing. When something is not right, it will give an indication, which can sometimes be in the form of a slight discharge. If this persists, you should consult a doctor. Make sure that your underwear is not too tight. It will also be helpful to use *Molkosan* in a hip bath. *Echinacea* can be valuable; taking *Echinaforce* (twenty drops three times a day) will be of great assistance. It would also be a good idea to try to read my books *Menstrual and Premenstrual Tension* and *Menopause,* both of which give a lot of worthwhile advice.

To have a healthy sex life does not always mean having a good sex life. To be able to enjoy sex to the full, it is vital to be sensible in your choice of sexual partner so as to avoid the risk of contracting sexually transmitted diseases, and not to 'sleep around' or have casual sex. If in any doubt whatsoever, it is imperative not to engage in unprotected sex. The most sensitive areas in the human body are the rectum, the bladder, the anus, the penis, the urethra and the testicles in men and, in women, the womb, the cervix, the rectum, the bladder and the vagina. Infections in these areas can often be a consequence of certain sexual acts. As I have mentioned, it is crucial that you are careful in your choice of sexual partner, as failing to do so could result in HIV, hepatitis B, gonorrhoea and syphilis. It is therefore essential to consult a doctor if you have any unusual symptoms, and not to take any risks.

A lady who consulted me some time ago reminded me of the many times I have come across this next problem with patients. She experienced a nasty burning pain during sexual intercourse. This is one of the symptoms of vulvitis, a particularly unpleasant inflammation which is basically a vaginal fungal condition. The medical terminology for this problem is vulvar vestibulitis syndrome. One has to be very vigilant with this condition to ensure that it is brought under control quickly, otherwise it might lead to more extensive problems. Most people think of this as a venereal disease, but its origin is often hormonal, hereditary or a problem in the autoimmune system.

There are some excellent natural remedies available to help this, such as *Yeast Balance* from Enzymatic, *Echinaforce* and *Nature-C*, a natural vitamin C from A. Vogel. In addition, sometimes a vitamin A supplement can help. There is also a very good cream that can be used, called *Chickweed Ointment,* from Abbots of Leigh. It is possible that this condition might also affect one's partner, whereby the pleasure of sex can be greatly restricted. If this is the case, then using a lubricating jelly, which you can buy from any chemist, could help. If this problem persists, then it may be useful to use *Calendula Ointment* or *Tea Tree Ointment* topically or some diluted *Molkosan.*

Vulvitis can develop as a result of an allergy or chemical irritation caused by such things as feminine deodorant sprays, scented soap or bubble bath. These are therefore best avoided, as they can make the problem worse. Daily cleansing with unperfumed soap, adequate rinsing and thorough drying of the genital area is one of the best ways to alleviate the burning and itching symptoms. It may also be useful to carry out some pelvic-floor exercises. The problem can be extremely painful and very unpleasant; it is a condition that doesn't permit the sexual pleasure that one is hoping for. To get rid of it, I sometimes resort to the use of acupuncture. I would also advise the elimination of sugar from the diet, and with the help of acupuncture, this will take a lot of the pain away. It is also important to relax by carrying out some of the relaxation exercises that I have mentioned in previous chapters.

These conditions often result in the loss of sexual desire (libido) and can sometimes lead to the break-up of relationships. Whatever the sexual activities, they should be enjoyed to the full. Libido tends to wax and wane and there are periods in people's lives when they have little desire for sex. It is normally a temporary phase and not a disaster. I often see this when treating patients with menstrual and premenstrual tension. The female partner may feel at certain times in the month that she has no desire for sex or intimacy whatsoever or that she 'can't be bothered'. I sometimes see women who are reduced to tears because their libido has completely gone, and they ask what can be done. Luckily, there are some very valuable remedies, such as *Female Balance,* which will help tremendously with menstrual and premenstrual tension, together with *Mood Essence* and *Female Essence,* both flower essences which can do no harm whatsoever. If desire has completely gone, there is a remedy from America called *For Women* which basically instils a greater sexual appetite.

During menopause, we see too often that a woman totally loses interest in lovemaking, or even turns into a Jekyll-and-Hyde character. This can be due to a lack of progesterone or an imbalance in oestrogen, in which case it will be beneficial to try some aromatherapy or reflexology in order to give the endocrine system a boost, and also to take a few remedies to produce extra vital oestrogen, or whatever else is lacking. *Female Essence,* together with *Phytogen* (an excellent product from Hadley Wood Healthcare), is often the answer.

I still think that some of the best research done in this day and age was that carried out into a natural progesterone. The result was a product called *Naturone,* which is completely natural and creates a balance in oestrogen and progesterone. This remedy is made from virgin macadamia oil, avocado oil, marula oil (which is antibacterial), vitamin E (as an antioxidant), ceto-stearyl alcohol (which is a vegetable-based emulsifier), glycerol (of vegetable origin), grapefruit extract (a natural preservative) and deionised water. This definitely does not contain progestins, animal derivatives, mineral oils, oestrogenic compounds, colourants or chemical preservatives.

In situations where there is a hormonal imbalance, menstrual or premenstrual tensions or menopausal influence, we often find patients suffering from mild depression, mood swings, panic attacks, sleeping problems, bloating, perimenopausal weight gain, irregular menstrual cycle, mastitis, fibroids, increased risk of breast cancer and other oestrogen cancers, fibrocystic breast disease, fertility problems, water retention, decreased libido, increased risk of stroke and heart disease, thinning skin, chronic fatigue, hypertension and high blood pressure, migraine headaches caused by the onset of osteoporosis and other menopausal complaints. Where there is a progesterone imbalance, *Naturone* will restore this.

It is quite interesting to note that this product is also a great help for Alzheimer's, aggression, allergies, alcoholism, autoimmune disease, arthritic pain and swelling, hypoglycaemia, hyperglycaemia, cancer, constipation, epilepsy, eye problems, polycystic ovaries, endometriosis, skin disorders, acne, cracked heels, bruising, thyroid problems and urinary tract infections. In fact, one could say it can treat everything! I have been amazed for some time at the results I have achieved from recommending this product. It is also extremely easy to use, as it can be applied to the skin for rapid absorption and it is relatively inexpensive. Having used this product in combination with the other remedies I have mentioned, I have been encouraged by the radical improvements made by many patients. Not only does the patient's sexual appetite improve but in addition the treatment often helps with many other health problems. Many patients who have consulted me on these matters have obtained great benefit from its use.

I frequently see how devastated men can become when they

experience problems with impotence (an inability to achieve or sustain an erection for satisfactory sexual activity). They often admit to me that they even want to end their lives. I am well aware that this condition may make men feel inadequate, even embarrassed or ashamed, because they cannot perform like other men. I usually have a long chat with them and try to get them to understand that sex is not the most important thing in life and certainly not in a relationship. It is much more important in a genuine relationship for a couple to be on the same wavelength and, this being the case, the sexual side will often correct itself. However, a lot of men are very impatient to get a quick result, which is impossible. In this situation, we are dealing with the finest material on earth – the individual human being – and the minute we tell the brain that we cannot do something, it will just not work – even the slightest hesitation will have an adverse effect.

There are, however, wonderful things that can help. An excellent remedy which is often successful in dealing with erection problems is *Masculex,* from Enzymatic. It contains extracts of muira puama, Mexican damiana and ginkgo biloba. Muira puama, an extract from a plant in the Amazon region of South America, is widely used as a powerful aphrodisiac, nerve stimulant, tonic and cure for rheumatism and muscle paralysis. Research indicates that it is one of the best herbs for erectile dysfunction or lack of libido. Recent studies have validated its safety and effectiveness in improving libido and treating sexual dysfunction in some patients. At the Institute of Sexology in Paris, muira puama has been the subject of three published clinical studies conducted by Dr Jacques Waynberg, one of the world's foremost authorities on sexual function and author of ten books on the subject. The first study comprised 262 men complaining of lack of sexual desire or inability to attain or maintain an erection. The result, after 2 weeks, was that 62 per cent of patients with loss of libido rated the treatment as having a dynamic effect, while 52 per cent of those with erectile dysfunction rated the treatment as beneficial. Dr Waynberg's second study focused on sexual difficulties associated with asthenia, a deficiency state characterised by fatigue, loss of strength or debility. The study consisted of 100 men over 18 years of age who complained of impotence, loss of libido, or both. A total of 94 men completed the study. Muira puama treatment led to significantly increased frequency of intercourse for 66 per cent of participants. Of the 46 men who complained of loss of desire, 70 per cent reported intensification of libido. The stability of erection during intercourse was restored in 55 per cent of patients, and 66 per cent of men reported a reduction in fatigue. Other beneficial effects included improvement in sleep and morning erections.

Treatment with muira puama was much more effective in cases with less psychosomatic involvement. Of the 26 men diagnosed with common sexual asthenia without noticeable sign of psychosomatic disorder, the treatment was effective for asthenia in 100 per cent of cases, for lack of libido in 85 per cent of cases and for inability to obtain an erection in 90 per cent of cases. The latter finding confirms the broad tonic action of muira puama in conditions of fatigue and stress-related sexual dysfunction. Since muira puama is not an artificial stimulant, it fortifies the system over a period of time. Some men report increased vitality within two weeks, while the full effects build over several weeks.

Waynberg noted that his toxicology studies and observations corroborated the conclusions of the scientific literature on the absence of toxicity in muira puama, which is well tolerated by men in generally good health. An early French study found muira puama to be effective in gastrointestinal and circulatory asthenia as well as impotence. Three of the most respected scientific authorities on medical herbalism recommend muira puama in their published works. James Duke Ph.D., chief of the United States Department of Agriculture's medical plant laboratory, and renowned naturopath Michael Murray recommend muira puama for erectile dysfunction or lack of libido. Presently, the mechanism of action in muira puama is unknown. From the information available, it appears that it works by enhancing both psychological and physical aspects of sexual function.

Damiana (*Turnera diffusa*), another of the ingredients of *Masculex*, is known to have been used as an aphrodisiac in the ancient Mayan civilisation, and a Spanish missionary first reported that the Mexican Indians made a drink from the damiana leaves, added sugar and drank it for its purported power to enhance lovemaking. Damiana has a long history of use in traditional herbal medicine throughout the world. It is thought to act as an aphrodisiac, antidepressant, tonic, diuretic, cough suppressant and mild laxative. It has been used for such conditions as depression, anxiety, sexual inadequacy, debility, bed-wetting, menstrual irregularities, gastric ulcers and constipation. In Mexico, the plant is also taken in cases of asthma, bronchitis, diabetes, dysentery, dyspepsia, headaches, nephrosis, neurosis, paralysis, spermatorrhoea, stomachache and syphilis. Its traditional uses include: as a male and female sexual stimulant used to treat erectile dysfunction and anorgasmia; to tone, balance and strengthen the central nervous system and for emotional stress, depression and anxiety; as a general hormonal balancer; for nervous stomach, colic and dyspepsia; and for mood disorders (hypochondria, obsessive-compulsive disorder, neurosis, paranoia etc.). Its only downside is that it may reduce the absorption of iron.

Sometimes the inclusion of extra vitamin E in the diet will help, and if there is a total lack of erection, then taking one or two capsules of *Man Power* from Michael's daily will often do a better job than Viagra. One should try not to worry, as this can prolong the problem.

For some time now I have been concerned about the increased incidence of men consulting me with Peyronie's disease. The cause of this disease is unknown, but it appears to have increased more during the last five years than in all the years I have been in practice. It is a dysplasia of the cavernous sheaths, consisting of a fibrous thickening and contracture of the investing fascia of the corpora, not unlike Dupuytren's contracture. The contracture can reduce the flexibility of the penis, causing pain and forcing it to bend or arc during erection, making sexual intercourse painful or almost impossible. In such cases, I have found ultrasonic treatment to be beneficial. The sexual problems that result from this condition can disrupt a couple's physical and emotional relationship and lead to lowered self-esteem in the man. I have had a long search to find a way of helping patients with this particular condition, as it is basically a mechanical problem and because doctors are not keen to operate. I have found that a German remedy called *Araniforce* gives good results together with *Osteo Factors* from Michael's. These have benefited a number of patients who have suffered from this disease and its consequences for a long time.

In cases of sexual dysfunction, I have seen both men and women becoming very uptight and frustrated. It may be useful to read some of the many books available for guidance on this subject. The sexual organs are easily disturbed. If you become worried and miserable about it, this can cause additional stress and anxiety. It is therefore best to try to relax about it as much as possible and to be positive. If you find the matter too distressing, try not to dwell on it. Speak to your partner about any fears you may have and then take positive steps to deal with them. Whatever feelings come over us, whatever emotions might emerge, we all have to learn to accept them. In order to start the healing process, once we accept ourselves, we can then begin to love ourselves and our relationships much more.

If there is an obstacle in your life, it is important to sit down and ask yourself what the most important thing in your life is and what you can do to change. Life is all about relationships. A close, loving relationship is a question of giving and receiving the energy that is all around us. As I have mentioned in several of my books, when I worked in China I was taught three important things – to *look,* to *listen* and to *feel.* Look at the situation objectively and look at what might be happening in your life or what the disturbance is, listen to your inner self, sit down, relax and meditate, and then feel the vibrations around you, because often a small vibratory disturbance can lead to a great deal of misfortune. As I have said in this chapter, where we deal with the finest material on earth, we have to be very sensitive.

A young, elegant couple consulted me recently. I could sense they felt uneasy as they asked me what they could do about the man's condition. He had been diagnosed with type 2 diabetes about two years earlier. He had coped with that fairly well, but because his blood sugar was very high, he had been prescribed strong medication to get this under control. Unfortunately, this affected his sexual performance. This was putting a strain on their close relationship, although his wife was very understanding. They felt he was too young for Viagra, and asked if there were any other possibilities. I asked him about his diabetes, which he now had under control. We then had a long discussion about his dietary management. I recommended a remedy I use regularly for diabetics called *Daily Choice for Glucose Regulation,* which was extremely helpful and, to increase his sexual performance, I recommended vitamin E (one capsule of 400 units twice daily), one *Man Power* capsule to be taken in the morning and, twice daily, one capsule of *Masculex,* together with fifteen drops of *Ginkgo biloba* twice daily. This combination worked within two to three weeks, and at their next visit two months later, they were one of the happiest couples I have ever met, telling me how wonderful everything was.

I remember a fairly young man who consulted me. He had been an alcoholic and a drug addict and his sexual desire had totally gone. This upset him greatly, but luckily he had managed to stop both drinking and drug abuse. Fortunately for him, the damage caused had not been too severe, but it took almost five months before some improvement was noticed. He has now, fortunately, returned to normal.

Sadly, this is not always the case. Sometimes stronger remedies have to be taken, or in some instances, if the damage is too severe, sexual desire might not return at all. However, even after all these years in practice, I never cease to be amazed. Another couple who consulted me had, for some unknown reason, both lost all interest in sex. The lady thought that in her case it might have been due to menstrual tension, but the man did not know why he had lost all interest. As they were keen to restore their relationship, they were prepared to do anything to remedy the situation. At the outset, I felt this would be a difficult problem to solve. I tried a few things, but they did not work. I then asked them both to try magnetic therapy, which is widely recommended in this book. It was almost unbelievable how, after a few months, both of them got a terrific lift and things started to return to normal. Not only were they delighted about this, but they also felt that their energy had improved overall. As I said earlier, I had been sceptical for a long time about this form of treatment, but I have to admit that it works, although differently from other forms of treatment. It is actually very difficult to explain how it does work, and in this case I was left without an explanation, although I knew that the magnetic treatment had restored their energies.

I was once asked at a medical convention how magnetic therapy works. Although we want to know about everything in black and white and have it scientifically explained, this is not always possible. I feel that we have only scratched the surface of what energy really is, but I believe it to be the future of medicine. At this particular meeting, I was asked several times to try to give an explanation, which I found very difficult. One particular professor kept pressing me for answers, so I put the ball back in his court by asking him if he could tell me how conception really works.

There are explanations for many things, but some still mystify me, as I often see in my work with acupuncture, which I sometimes use in cases of sexual difficulties or problems which could have a devastating effect on someone's sex life. I still find it intriguing how, around 5,000 to 6,000 years ago, the ancient Chinese realised that certain points in the body could restore that particular energy, and I find it even more difficult to give an explanation for it. Sometimes I concur with colleagues who say that it doesn't matter how it works as long as it does. That too is difficult to accept, yet when people tell me how happy they are when certain problems have disappeared purely by the use of simple acupuncture treatment, I cannot feel unhappy about it. As one can see, there are many ways to help with sexual problems, to restore a couple's relationship and to achieve the best for sexual health.

CHAPTER ELEVEN

What to Do About Infertility

One evening last year, I gave a lecture attended by between 5,000 and 6,000 people. The hall was full, and, luckily, my talk went well. I usually speak for about an hour and then give the audience an opportunity to put questions to me. When it came to that moment in the proceedings, a lady stood up and said that she wanted to thank me for making her pregnant! Well, as the packed hall looked up at me and booed, I realised I had a lot of explaining to do. To cut a long story short, this lady and her husband had consulted me quite some time ago, after trying for a baby for 17 years. They desperately wanted a child. The problem lay with the husband and it actually took very little intervention to sort things out. She then became pregnant and gave birth to twins. After I had clarified this to the audience, they were satisfied.

It sometimes takes only a minor adjustment when pregnancy seems impossible, as was the case with this couple. The lady was perfectly healthy, but her husband had developed mumps as a child, a disease which can result in a man being sterile. Because of this man's childhood illness, there were quite a lot of miasmas – leftovers from former inflammation, viruses or infections – in his system, which I was able to remove using homoeopathy. Curing like with like is very important and once the miasmas are out of the system, which can take several stages of treatment, there is much that can be done. If there is something in the body that is not right, you should do everything in your power to eliminate it before it causes further problems. After the miasmas were out of his system, things turned out well, hence this lady bursting to tell everyone that, through my help, she became pregnant.

I have made it possible for many childless couples in the world to finally have the baby they so desperately desire. Even when they have almost given up hope, it is surprising how, often by making only a few small adjustments, conception can become possible. Sometimes it just needs the right diagnosis at the right time to get to the bottom of the problem, which can then be dealt with.

Infertility can be a big problem, but there are remedies that can help. To understand the problem, I would like to explain a little bit about fertility.

Going away together after marriage is a very old custom. In the Middle Ages, when a man wanted a child, he often abducted a woman and went into hiding with her during a phase of the moon (for about a month). During this time, it was the custom that every day both of them should drink some honeyed wine (mead), which was said to improve fertility. Mead was a fermented mixture of honey, water and fruit juices, and it is thought that this was the first alcoholic drink people produced.

We know now that honey contains many different vitamins, minerals, enzymes, hormones and other important substances, and therefore it seems to be quite possible that honey increases fertility. At the same time, a reluctant bride, under the influence of the light alcohol content of honeyed wine, became more pliable. For the same reason, a little wine during the honeymoon will help newlyweds to relax together. However, although a little wine does not hurt, a couple should definitely not touch hard alcoholic drinks if they are trying to conceive.

These days, most people go on honeymoon in order to relax, to get to know one another more intimately, to have a lovely holiday and to be happy. For some, though, the most important objective is to get away from other people and, if possible, start creating their first child. When planning a honeymoon, many people choose to go on a cruise or to a nice hotel in some big city they have always wanted to visit. Both choices are wrong if the couple plans to start a family. The original idea of a honeymoon is to get away from people and to relax. Big cities and cruises may be fine for a normal holiday, but for a couple who want to conceive they are the wrong choice. On cruises and in big cities, relaxation is not possible.

Many cultures today still have ritualistic celebrations in homage to the gods of fertility. In olden times, the only way to ensure that one's line survived was to have many children, and so the fertility of human beings has always been very important.

Nature is very wise. When people are not healthy, it will be very difficult or even impossible for them to have a baby. Causes of infertility include a wide range of physical, emotional and environmental factors. The 'seeds' of some men are too weak or the sperm count is too low. Some women will not be able to accept the sperm of the man because of ovulation dysfunction. This can be due to poor nutrition, hormonal imbalance, ovarian cysts, an abnormal uterus, a history of pelvic inflammatory diseases or other problems.

Not long ago, there was an article in the Austrian newspaper *Die Presse* which was headed 'Sperm quality is going down continuously'. It said, 'Because of chemical pollution, according to university professor

Dr Walter Ludvik, the sperm quality in men has decreased by 30 per cent during the last three decades.' For this, the professor blames the destruction of the environment, exhaust fumes, heavy metals (such as lead), fertilisers, preservatives and pesticides. People take in all these toxins with their daily nutrition and when they use polluted water for drinking and cooking.

Newsweek recently reported that since 1938 the average sperm count had decreased by 50 per cent and that during the same period the number of patients suffering from cancer of the prostate had trebled. In 1940, it was estimated that about 7 million American men suffered from erectile dysfunction. Now the estimate is between 15 and 25 million, and when partial impotence is included this goes up to about 30 million. In Europe, the estimates are also pretty high.

Fertility and infertility are emotional issues that can be difficult for a couple to face and openly discuss with each other. For many couples, fertility is something they take for granted and they are often surprised when the woman does not become pregnant as soon as they start trying for a baby. However, many couples find they are unable to conceive straight away and this can put their relationship under immense pressure. Overall, around one in six couples seek help and advice when they experience difficulties in conceiving. In such cases, many months of fruitless attempts can feel like an eternity. As I tell a lot of unhappy couples, it only needs one active sperm and one tiny egg to become pregnant, but, nevertheless, there are many obstacles that can stand in the way of this wonderful match between male and female.

Female Reproductive Factors from Michael's has proved to be helpful for many patients who have had difficulties conceiving. It addresses specific nutrients that aid normal conception and carrying to full term while supporting the entire female hormonal system, creating optimal conditions for a very healthy conception and pregnancy. It contains vitamin C and bioflavonoids for healthy ovaries and ovum, with the herbs Mexican wild yam and unicorn root traditionally used by women of child-bearing age for support.

To increase male fertility, improving sperm health, count and motility, or ability to swim against the current, while promoting a strong and healthy conception and embryo, it would be helpful to try a formula called *Male Reproductive Factors* from Michael's or *Doctor's Choice for Men* from Enzymatic, which contains herbal extracts including muira puama to improve libido and sexual function, together with ginseng to help support healthy testosterone levels. It is necessary to try to relax more and to have a positive approach.

Sometimes a very specific problem can be identified, as I discovered with one lady who had tried for several years to become pregnant. As we discussed her medical history in detail, it transpired that she had consulted many practitioners before coming to see me. Our Vegacheck machine indicated that she was extremely deficient in vitamin E. One has to be careful to administer vitamin E at the correct dosages. Vitamin E, often called 'the fertility vitamin', was appropriate for her. Although she had previously undergone extensive tests, nobody had discovered the real reason for her inability to conceive. It was not until I carried out tests using the machine that this became apparent. Vitamin E influences the development and functioning of muscles and prevents muscle degeneration. If there are any disturbances because of a lack of vitamin E, then it is important that this is administered with professional guidance.

I often ask myself how much we really know about vitamin E. From experience, we know it increases energy and vitality, but it was partly chance, as well as acute observation and clear, logical thinking, that led us to the discoveries that serve us today of the benefits we obtain from vitamin E when it is administered properly. It can be most useful in infertility cases, as with this patient, who, amazingly, became pregnant within two months. I was satisfied for her to keep taking this supplement for a while to reduce the risk of miscarriage. She gave birth to a lovely baby, whose photograph is proudly displayed among the collection of photographs of those babies whose conception I have helped to make possible.

Many women who have been unable to conceive because of endometriosis have found great hope in a remedy called *Endobrit* that was created almost by accident by a homoeopathic doctor in Australia. She discovered that a particular combination of several homoeopathic remedies gave tremendous results in women suffering from endometriosis and other infertility problems. Following thorough research, it is now available on the British market.

I was so pleased the other day when I met a lady in the street who proudly showed me her baby. Some time previously, I had prescribed a few simple remedies for her, such as *Endobrit,* vitamin E and *Female Reproductive Factors.* I also recommended that both her husband and she should have some reflexology and aromatherapy, which are of great benefit. The end result was another desperately wanted baby.

One can appreciate that when a couple yearn for a baby, they will do everything they possibly can, so it is understandable in such instances that both partners can have feelings of inadequacy. Conception is a remarkably complex process, and the prospect of being infertile can have a devastating impact on the well-being of both men and women. The problem could be caused by a hormone deficiency or, as is often the case, circulatory problems. It is therefore worthwhile checking that the blood circulation is in order. I came across such a case when I was working in the United States. It was arranged that I would lecture in three states during my visit. On this particular day, I had to catch two flights and during the morning I had a lot of appointments. I was consulting at a large health store, where I offered free advice for two hours. An attractive young couple came up to me, both in tears, and told me that every avenue had been investigated – his sperm count and motility were normal, and she was reported to be fine as well. Unexplained infertility was the reason given by the doctors they saw. 'Unexplained infertility' is the phrase used when a couple have been investigated and all the test results are normal.

Anyway, we chatted for a while and, because my selection of medicines was low in that particular place and I wanted to do my best to help them, by chance I asked her if she had any circulatory problems. She told me that she had varicose veins and haemorrhoids, which are clear indications that such problems exist. When I looked into her eyes, I could see that her body was also low in calcium. Luckily, the store had *Ginkgo biloba, Aesculus* and *Urticalcin,* all of which I prescribed for her. Sometimes, in places where I have been faced with the problem of certain remedies being unavailable and have had to concoct a combination of remedies, I have been amazed by their success.

Three months later, in Scotland, I received a letter from her telling me that she was pregnant but that she was terrified of losing the baby. I wrote back, advising her to take *Prenatal Formula* from Enzymatic, which I knew was available in the United States. I asked her to try to get hold of some as soon as possible and to let me know how things progressed. Believe it or not, the outcome was a beautiful baby who arrived exactly on its due date. Five years later, I visited that same store with some colleagues. Out of the blue, this same charming lady came up and hugged me tightly to thank me. She told me she was now the proud mother of three beautiful children and wondered if there was any link between her conceiving and taking *Ginkgo biloba.*

It may all look easy, but it certainly isn't. The fact remains that good blood circulation and proper nutrition (which I advised her about) did indeed help her over the first hurdles to becoming pregnant. I have kept in contact with this couple over the years, and it has been heart-warming to witness the immense happiness that I have brought into their lives. In fact, this lady had earlier told me that she had been contemplating divorce because her inability to conceive had put a great strain on her relationship with her husband. It is wonderful to see how much can be achieved with so little, providing the problem is tackled in the correct manner.

On another occasion, I was consulted by an attractive young lady who was a bag of nerves. She sat before me, shivering and shaking, until finally I managed to prise out of her that she was on Prozac and different tranquillisers and still wanted to get pregnant. I said that the first thing to do was to treat her nervous system sensibly to calm her down, and with some effective homoeopathic and herbal remedies, I managed to settle her down significantly and eliminate a lot of the toxic material in her body. As her nervous system began to improve, she realised there was a better world beyond Prozac. She had been married for eight years and was almost suicidal at the thought of not being able to conceive, all simply due to nerves. It is necessary to really relax in order to get the whole body back in tune. We managed this with the use of reflexology and aromatherapy. Miraculously, she became pregnant, and brought a beautiful son into the world, whose photograph, again, is displayed among the collection of those of babies I have been responsible for. These photographs take pride of place in my room and are a reminder of the little miracles that can happen. This woman and her husband are now the proud parents of three children. As a result of getting her nervous condition under control and saying goodbye to all the depression that she had, she is now extremely happy.

Alas, these stories do not always have a happy ending. I shall never forget a young man who tearfully told me he was convinced he was to blame for the fact that his wife had not become pregnant. Undeniably, he had a very low sperm count with no motility and had also had quite a number of illnesses. With sensitivity, I explained to him that the chances were slim but that I would do everything I possibly could to help him. Sadly, he never returned, and about two months later, he tragically hanged himself. The thought that he couldn't produce a baby led him to a point where he couldn't face life any longer, and, although he had a very understanding wife, he could no longer cope with the situation.

Treating infertility sometimes requires us to explain the apparently inexplicable. As I so often say, conception is such a complex system that it needs to be carefully dealt with. It is amazing to think of the many problems that can be overcome by giving nature a helping hand. One thing is for sure, as there are many things that are needed to enable this particular system to flourish, every avenue should be carefully investigated and any problems dealt with appropriately. It can be very difficult for a physician to find out the actual reason for infertility. The problem can frequently be stress related or due to an unhealthy lifestyle, and in such cases it can be remedied. Often, when both partners have changed their eating and living habits, in due course the woman will become pregnant. I have seen this happen even in the case of couples who had given up all hope.

I still remember the day a Greek lady came to see me. She and her husband had been married for over six years. They were hoping to have a child and both had seen several specialists. These physicians had conducted many tests, but there seemed to be nothing really wrong and their reproductive organs were healthy. They were told that it was probably just a question of too much stress and that they should try to relax more and enjoy life. Their last physician recommended that if this brought no results, they should see a psychiatrist! When she came to see me, this lady was quite desperate. She was not so young any more and soon it would be too late for her to have a child.

I spoke to her for a long time and enquired about their eating and living habits. It turned out that they ate at a snack bar twice a week and, at home, they often ate ready meals. Both had a lack of fresh vegetables in their diet and they never ate wholemeal bread, cereal or other such things. The lady told me that when she and her husband were engaged, they often used to go hiking or swimming, but since their marriage they hardly did any exercise or sports and only seldom went for a walk. I recommended that they take up these good habits again. Also, I urged that from then on they eat more home-made, fresh and wholesome food.

They both had a hair test done, and when a week later the results of this test came back, it turned out that both of them were lacking certain vitamins and minerals, which I prescribed in high doses. The lady suffered from toxic quantities of copper and mercury, and therefore it was no wonder that she could not conceive. I prescribed a homoeopathic remedy that would help to eliminate these toxins from her body.

After two months, the couple came to see me again. They were very happy and thanked me profusely, as the lady was now expecting their first child. The only problem for me was the fact that thereafter my office resembled a meeting place for Greek ladies who wanted to have children!

Modern food is lacking in many nutrients needed by our future citizens, and it would be good if young couples who were unable to procreate after a couple of years of trying had a hair test done in order to find out what vitamins or minerals are lacking. Hair tests are much more reliable than blood tests. This is due to the fact that the composition of the blood changes every so often. Hair taken from the neck of the person in question will indicate any lack of nutrients. Also, any accumulation of toxins will be revealed. Some toxins, especially from certain heavy metals or medicines, can cause health problems that prevent conception. Our modern world is full of toxins, and almost each day new and dangerous poisons are being used in industry or added to our food.

Men have their own biochemical problems. Typically, men are short of zinc. Zinc is the controlling element for male sexuality because it regulates testosterone levels. Testosterone levels dictate a man's (and a woman's) sexual appetite, his physical stamina and his sperm count. Low zinc levels also affect the sperm's motility. Normal zinc levels improve all of these. Old wives' tales about oysters being a great aphrodisiac are scientifically correct. Oysters are loaded with zinc. They are great for men wanting to make babies. Other foods high in zinc are lean beef, crab, eggs, sunflower seeds, trout and wheat bran.

Deficiencies are often easy to fix because if they are not too serious, one can simply eat more of the necessary foods and take the necessary supplements. Toxicity is a bigger problem. It may take a year to effectively deal with extreme toxicity. In these circumstances, toxins are usually lodged in every body cell. However, eating the right foods can naturally speed things up. The film star Sophia Loren suffered from this problem. After many years trying for a baby, it was eventually discovered that she had extremely high copper levels. Happily, she conceived shortly after the condition was treated.

Although our body needs a small amount of copper in order to stay healthy, copper imbalance seems to be a major cause of unexplained infertility. We know that the brain controls fertility in both men and women, and in order to function correctly, it needs some copper. However, too much has exactly the opposite effect. The copper/zinc ratio in your body regulates ovulation. If there is too much copper and too little zinc, a woman's fertility can be compromised. The imbalance can cause tumours and cysts to grow in the body, making it difficult to conceive. If a woman whose body contains too much copper does have a baby, there may be birth defects and the brain development of the baby may be adversely affected. Copper is not only found in water pipes and kitchenware but also in birth-control pills.

This is only one example of the complicated interaction of substances in our body. Being aware of all these things is vital if you want to conceive a healthy and happy baby. However, the intuitive understanding of a loving mother once the baby is born can be even more important.

While preparing this chapter, I couldn't help smiling as my thoughts turned to an elderly Scottish lady who came to see me. I had finished part of this chapter earlier that very morning and was particularly busy in the clinic when she arrived. She was extremely unsteady on her feet, so I helped her to a chair in my consulting room before taking care of some patients in the treatment room. As I was so absorbed in other things, I had almost forgotten that she was waiting to see me. As I returned to the consulting room, she was sitting clutching her handbag on her lap and studying my family photograph on the wall behind my desk. In a lovely Scottish accent, she asked me if these were all my children. I explained that the portrait showed my four daughters and ten grandchildren. I don't think she realised what she then said, but it made me smile for the remainder of the day. In a shaky voice, she said, 'My, my. Isn't it wonderful to see what a wee man like you is capable of.' Not only did this make me smile, but it reminded me once more what a great wonder conception is. I have the greatest compassion for women and men who try so hard to have their lives enriched by the miracle of birth. That is what life is all about and, as a father and grandfather, I shall always do my best to help wherever I can.

CHAPTER TWELVE

A Life Full of Health, Happiness and Vitality

Health is a wonderful thing. When you are healthy, you wake up in the morning and you look forward to the coming day. Life is a wonderful adventure, always worthwhile, even if sometimes we know sorrow and pain.

Health means that we enjoy life and that we can cope with many daily problems without being beaten down by them. When you are really healthy, you are like a jack-in-the-box: you might be pushed down, but you always spring up again. Health means to be happy, to enjoy your work and to love your family and friends. Health means that you have a well-balanced, kind personality. Health can give happiness and contentment; but when health is lost, living can be hell.

When our grandparents tell us stories about the good old times, when the sky was bluer, the water clearer and the people healthier, we do not believe them. Of course, we will accept the first two statements. We know that the air was cleaner and the water less polluted, but to believe that people were healthier is, of course, wishful thinking. We know that people died younger, that many babies did not live long and that there were terrible epidemics such as smallpox, typhus and tuberculosis that killed thousands of people. Now, thanks to progress and many new medicines, people live longer, most babies stay alive and those terrible epidemics have disappeared.

We let the older generation talk and we listen politely – we know better! But do we really know better? Why should the older generation be so right about their first statements and so completely wrong about the last one? To know the real truth about this, we should go much deeper into these problems. We should learn about health and about humankind, and only then might we be able to judge.

Millions of years ago, when the earth was still covered by dense woods, there were all kinds of different animals. Many apes lived in the trees, and when the woods became less dense and less food was to be found, some of these apes descended from the trees. They walked on their hind legs and they ate whatever they could find: small insects, worms, fruits, roots, wild berries and many more things. These apes became stronger and more intelligent. They started to hunt in groups and were able to catch young or small animals. The organs of these animals, like the heart and the liver, were a particular delicacy for them. Even nowadays, apes love to eat some kinds of meat if they can get them. In the wilds of Africa, you can see groups of big apes hunting down little impalas (a kind of antelope) and giving the livers to their young ones.

The first human beings also lived in this way. They hunted in groups and caught fish from the rivers and the sea by many ingenious means. The inner parts of these animals were a special treat for them, and they also used the fats and oils, which served many purposes. Furthermore, they lived on roots and grasses, on herbs, fruits and berries. Many tribes ate birds and eggs, insects and ants. Human beings always loved sweet things like honey. People who lived near the sea ate all kinds of seaweed, oysters, mussels and other products of the sea.

It was a hard life, and it was not always easy to find food. The men often had to run long distances in order to hunt down animals and the women of the tribe walked for hours to find the roots, the fruits and the different herbs they used. In times of scarcity, the whole tribe would often move to other surroundings. If they were hungry or weak, they knew to find special herbs, which, we know now, contained a very high percentage of certain vitamins and minerals. Sometimes they were almost starving by our standards, but the little food they found contained an exceptionally high quality of the essential building materials needed for health. When hungry times were over, their strength recovered quickly.

Expecting or nursing mothers, young, old or weak people received special foods, such as liver, heart, particular herbs, milk and blood, to make them strong. Before they married, young people were given certain herbs and extra portions of food. Each tribe had its own secret recipes. These people knew much more about the prevention of diseases than we do in our civilised countries, and they practised what they knew.

Of course, especially in the warm tropical countries, there were many dangers to human health, but primitive people could resist those very well and their numbers even multiplied. Only the very weak ones were destroyed. Most people died in hunting and fishing accidents or from old age, but, unlike old people who live in our wonderful modern world, they never knew the immense tragedy of seemingly endless suffering.

They had strong and elastic bones, which did not break easily, and those bones became harder and stronger as people became older because they always had great quantities of calcium, magnesium and other minerals in their daily food. Nowadays, people break their legs far too easily, and only animals living in their natural surroundings get stronger bones over the years. The chiefs and witch doctors of these people knew something about the setting of bones and they also knew what to do when someone was bitten by a poisonous insect or a snake – they were experts on many herbs. People who were ill took a rest and ate little or nothing until they felt better again. Their faith also helped them to recover and to overcome their problems.

In some parts of the world, the greatest problem was a lack of protein, resulting in 'big belly' sickness. But after meagre times came better times, and then all those problems disappeared. As long as people lived on natural food that had not been tampered with, they had an enormous amount of energy and strength, and a great resistance against diseases.

Human beings are part of nature, and so are plants and animals. Without them we would not be able to live. There are many known and many still unknown connections between plant, animal and human life. Although there seems to be a great difference between these three forms of life, all of them have the same basic requirements if they want to stay healthy and develop all their given qualities. They need air, soil and water. They need sunshine and rain. They need the right atmosphere in which to grow and, above all, they need the right food and to be able to discard their waste products.

If plants get the right kind of food, the right kind of humidity and sunshine, they stay healthy and all their leaves, flowers and fruits will fully develop. With animals, it is the same. Wild animals that eat the food which is meant for them have a great resistance against diseases. Their muscles and bones grow strong as they get older and their instincts become more acute. In the wilderness, it is very difficult to see the difference between old and young animals, even when one is quite nearby. The old animal jumps and runs almost as fast as the younger one. These animals die as a result of accidents or old age. When they feel that their strength is lessening and that their time is over, they leave the others to find a quiet spot where they can lie down and die in peace. This is the best way to die – not only for animals, but also for human beings!

In the severe cold of northern regions, in the dense wood of tropical climates, on the high mountains and in hidden, far-away corners of the earth, there still live people who are untouched by our Western civilisation. They live as their forefathers lived for many generations. The impression I have gained from my travels around the world – and from my talks with Alfred Vogel, who had been to some of the most remote places on earth researching his remedies – is that the lives of these people are not easy but that they are happy and cheerful and have comparatively few real problems.

The air they breathe is pure, the water they drink unpolluted and, above all, they eat food that is meant for them – fresh, unspoiled food that is often not even cooked. In some areas, the indigenous people often fast for a day or two after some special celebration. All they eat are the products of their own surroundings, of their own land. They live off their animals and their crops, from hunting and fishing and from whatever they can find in their natural environment. When they eat fish or meat, they also eat the organs, the glands, the blood and even some of the softer bones of these animals. They use their fat and oils for many purposes, especially in the high north. They use skins for their tents and their clothing, and as binding and sewing materials. Everything is used, nothing is wasted.

Fruits, wild vegetables, roots, different grains, seaweed, herbs and honey, if they can find it, are their daily fare. When they are thirsty, they drink water, plain juices or slightly fermented juices from different fruits or plants. In Africa, they use the milk of the coconut, and in Mexico, fermented cacti juices. Some domesticated animals give them milk and milk products.

All these people, in different places and climates of the earth, eat very different kinds of food, depending on their environment; but all of them eat natural, unpolluted food. They tend to have very healthy bodies and good bone structure. Colds, sinus troubles, allergies, constipation, headaches, diabetes or cancer are still unknown to them. There is no crime, there are no drugs and no modern diseases. Most people die from natural causes.

The daily food intake of these people provides them with about four to eight times as many vitamins, minerals, amino acids and other essentials as we get in a day. They have no doctors or dentists, but they know what to do in case of accidents or when people are sick. After disastrous weather conditions or a poor harvest, people are often hungry and some of them die, but the stronger ones stay alive and recover quickly when enough food is again available.

These people still exist in far-away places where civilisation has not yet invaded their peaceful life, but what happens when new airstrips are built or new shipping lines are created? When this happens, the shock and the impact of this sudden change to the life of primitive people can be so great that their entire way of living can be totally altered within a couple of weeks. Their whole normal existence is thrown out of focus. These people suddenly realise that there exists a completely different kind of life from their own. Only the very careful and the very strong characters will be able to resist all the new temptations.

Take, for example, the experience of the Navajo Indians in North America. 'Civilised' people came in their aeroplanes and in their boats. They brought many new and beautiful things with them: electricity and radios, new material and clothes, knowledge and books. They built roads and strong houses. They also brought food – all kinds of new food that looked good and tasted good, food which could be kept for weeks, months or even years, so that there was no need to be hungry in times of bad harvest or during the dry years. Many things had a nice, sweet taste, like honey. Children especially liked those sweet things and all the soft drinks. Their parents also liked the new food. Life was so much better now. They exchanged animal skins, pearls, meat or fish in return for beautiful white flour, white sugar, oil without a strong taste, sweets, chocolate and much tinned food. The children got popcorn, chewing gum, ice creams and many other wonderful things. Bakeries and convenience stores were installed where you could buy fluffy white bread, and when people had little time because there were so many new things to do, it was so easy just to open one of these nice little tins and heat its contents in a lovely new pan. They listened to the radio, looked at television and felt proud when they realised that now they had the same things as the rich people. Never before had they known how good life could be and how easy!

But there are two sides to every coin, and after a while some of the children started complaining of toothaches and cavities. These complaints had been very rare in the past. There were also other troubles which they had rarely seen before – people started to complain about headaches, colds, sinus troubles and allergies, and some of them were constantly tired. Formerly, they had been tired after hard work, very tired sometimes, but now they were tired before they even started work. They were listless and they became ill. Because of this, children could not go to school and grown-ups could not go to their work. They missed many working hours and things were left undone. Now they needed doctors and medical care, and civilisation provided those. It also brought in doctors and dentists, pharmacies and hospitals.

Now there was also crime. Never before had there been any real crime. When people did something wrong, they were punished by the elders, but seldom had there been any serious offence. People became nervous and did not trust each other any more. Gone were their happiness and their beautiful smiles. There was no real contentment any more. The wonders of civilisation were still there, but they had lost most of their glamour. People did not feel like working, they just wanted to rest and to enjoy all the new things which had changed their entire lives.

More and more money was spent on many objects which were not really needed. More and more money was used to cover all the cost of health care and to pay for the hours in which these sick people could not work. Their faces became smaller, their bone structure changed and the shapes of their bodies also altered. There was a great difference between the children who had been born before civilisation came and after that time. The children that were born later had smaller breasts and their bones were narrower. They could not breathe as well as the other children. Terrible diseases like TB started in those changed settlements. When the doctors got the TB under control with their newest medicines, other illnesses which were more difficult to control, like diabetes, started. Some people even got cancer. More and more people became ill and there were even some mental illnesses.

The 'wonders' of civilisation had done terrible harm. People had not known how difficult it was to accept the good things, but also to be aware of the bad things which came from far-away countries. On television, everything looked so very beautiful. How could it be that everything turned out so different? The price paid for 'civilisation' had been far too high.

In order to understand what happened to the health of these poor people, we have to learn something more about the human body and the causes of disease.

The human body is a masterpiece of nature. It is made out of all kinds of tissues, organs, glands and different body fluids, and all these things are made out of cells. Our entire body is one big mass of cells. All these cells have a certain lifespan, after which they have to be replaced by new cells. We have muscle cells, blood cells, the cells of the skin, of our glands and of our organs. Every one of these cells can stay healthy, do its work and fulfil its duty within our body as long as it gets the right food and can get rid of its waste products. The blood and other body fluids bring the food to the cells and also take away their waste. As long as our cells stay healthy, we feel fine and have no complaints.

Our body needs proteins, carbohydrates and different kinds of fat. It also needs vitamins, minerals, amino acids, enzymes, hormones and many other known and as-yet-unknown building materials. In our Western countries, we usually get enough proteins, carbohydrates and fat, but many vitamins and minerals which are essential for our health are almost entirely missing from our diet.

When our body cells do not get what they need, they cannot function properly any more and they become too weak to get rid of their own waste materials. When these waste materials accumulate in the cells, the cells suffocate in their own dirt, they become ill and many of them die. Millions and millions of cells make up the human body, but when many of them become ill and die before their time, the entire body suffers and is not healthy any more. All the body fluids are filled with these waste materials that are very toxic. Now, as these body fluids become more and more saturated, the body has to get rid of these dangerous toxins and there will be a reaction. Great pressure has been building up inside the body and what we call 'illness' is, in reality, a kind of explosion. With all its energy, the body pushes these dangerous toxins out before they can do any more harm. In cases where this toxic saturation of the body is not yet very serious, those reactions will be weak and we will get a cold or a headache. When the saturation is worse, the reaction will be much stronger and we might get bronchitis or measles, a kidney infection or some other serious problem.

All so-called 'diseases' are only the symptoms of a general toxification of the body, and these symptoms will be noticed first at the weakest places of that body and at the different emergency exits which were specially constructed for this purpose. For example, problems may arise at the nose, the ears, the anus or the vagina, or at the deeper-lying organs connected with these superficial tubes and organs. The body can also expel many of its toxins by way of perspiration and it can destroy them by a higher temperature. Everything possible is always done by nature to drive out all harmful substances, to clean the body and to rebuild health, and the less we interfere, the stronger we will be.

This pressure which is building up inside the human body has different causes. You know already that one of these causes is that our cells are not healthy any more because they do not get the nourishment they need. Why does the human cell need so many different materials and why can it not function just as well when some of them are missing? All things in nature are made according to very definite laws. The structure of human, animal or plant cells is more or less the same. When these cells are broken down, we see that they are all made from the same building materials and contain the same kind of waste products. All these cells can absorb parts of one another as their nourishment. Each piece of meat, each fruit and each vegetable has its own specific composition.

We know more or less what our different foods contain, but we don't know everything about them. Each of them has its own quantity of proteins, carbohydrates, minerals, vitamins, enzymes, amino acids, hormones and many other things. The natural composition of each kind of food is always the same. Each has its own special formula, and this formula is a secret of nature. No pharmaceutical chemist can ever imitate them, although they often think they can. There are far too many unknown factors and life can never be explained by or substituted with a chemical formula.

Now, every living cell can only accept parts of other cells as its food under the condition that their composition is complete. If something is missing, the absorption will be incomplete or cannot take place at all, in which case the cell gets only very little nourishment or no nourishment at all. When this happens regularly, our cells become weak. They cannot do their work properly, they become ill and many of them die.

Let me give you an example. If you are in need of a certain building material, let us say calcium, you can drink a glass of milk. Pure, fresh milk, as long as it is not boiled or tampered with in any other way, is a very good natural food. Now, in your body this milk will go towards the cells which need calcium, and the calcium from the milk will be absorbed together with the milk fat and its other ingredients. We do know that milk contains calcium, milk fat, magnesium, vitamin A and several other things, but there are probably many other materials in milk which we have not yet discovered and maybe never will.

According to the laws of nature, a particular group of certain ingredients always belongs together. If some of these are taken away or if they are exchanged for something else, this food loses its real value. If some mineral, for example, has been taken out of the milk by the process of evaporation or sterilisation, this milk is not a complete product any more. If you drink skimmed milk, which does not contain milk fat, only very little of the calcium this milk contains, or possibly none at all, can be absorbed by your body cells. Your body is not capable of absorbing only one ingredient if the other ingredients are missing. Now you can, for example, try to replace this milk fat by some other kind of fat which you consume at the same time as you drink the milk, but the absorption will never be as complete.

Nature has great wisdom. In nature, everything that belongs together is put together in exactly the right quantities, and this is the food meant for us human beings. We can absorb this kind of food easily. We can stay healthy and develop all our given talents. Some people think that they know the secrets of nature. They change our food and even try to make entirely artificial food. We are playing with fire. If we destroy nature, we ourselves will be destroyed eventually.

As a result of wrong ideas and also as a result of the complete lack of thinking by the majority of the public, it is almost impossible in our Western countries to find any food which has not been tampered with. Everyone likes food that tastes good and has a nice colour, and many people like to eat great quantities of food. We ask for this kind of food and our factories make it. They bleach and boil and press and colour our food until it is exactly to our liking, and we enjoy eating it; but it is devoid of most of its valuable ingredients.

Plants take all the minerals and other essentials which they need for their growth out of the earth, and they stay healthy unless they lack certain building materials or fluids. Animals that live in their natural surroundings will only eat the food which is meant for them. Instinctively, they know exactly what is right for them and what does them harm. Only some imprisoned or domesticated animals have to eat what is put before them. Because of 'love', the owners of pets get them used to all kinds of foods that are not good for them, and because of this, cats and dogs often get the same kinds of diseases as human beings, the same complaints as their masters.

Out of the same kind of 'love', you often give your friends exactly the kind of food that they should never eat if you want them to stay healthy. People put anything in their mouths that looks nice and tastes good. They do not have the slightest idea what is good for them. Grandparents, uncles and aunts give sweets to children because they 'love' them so much, but in doing this, they get them used to the kinds of foods which may eventually destroy their health. Those foods which have been altered so much that they do not have the slightest resemblance any more to the original food from which they are made cannot be absorbed by our body cells in the right way and are extremely dangerous to our health.

Even when we eat natural food, there is proof that only about half of the minerals contained in that food can be absorbed. Our cells can only work at a certain speed. Primitive people who live on natural food get between four and eight times as many minerals and other essential building materials as we do each day. Because of this, they have much more strength and a very great resistance against diseases.

When their valuable daily food is exchanged all of a sudden for food that is almost completely devoid of these materials, the shock is so enormous that almost overnight they change from healthy into unhealthy people. Of course, there are also some other reasons for the onset of all these new diseases, but the food factor is always the most obvious and important.

This complete change of life which happens so suddenly when primitive people come into contact with civilisation also happened to the people of our Western countries a few centuries ago. The only difference was that this change came more slowly, so slowly in fact that we did not realise the great impact this made upon our health, our bone structure, our character and our entire way of living. This so-called 'civilisation' changed our lives so much that we now call our countries 'the civilised countries'. If this is indeed something we can be proud of, it is nevertheless highly questionable in many respects.

After the early times of primitive life, when people started to use fire more and more for cooking their food, some essential parts of this food were destroyed by the heat and its digestion became more difficult. Many of the terrible diseases of the Middle Ages were caused in the first place by polluted drinking water and the indescribable dirt that was found everywhere. Later on, people paid a little more attention to their personal hygiene. But their food became more refined. They ate many sweet things and drank more alcoholic beverages. Also, some of those people were eating enormous quantities of food.

Each period had its special kind of diseases, which had their origin in the kinds of lives people led and in the food they consumed.

Poverty and lack of sanitation played an important role. But even if people did not live in a very healthy way, their food had not yet really been tampered with. Many weak children and old people died, but the people who stayed alive were fairly strong and healthy.

This went on for several centuries, until the first grain refineries were started. Now it was possible to eat real white bread made from wonderful white flour. At the same time, the best and most valuable parts of the grain were discarded. These parts were thrown away or used as animal feed. The same thing happened to sugar, to oil and to many other things which people ate every day. At about the same period, many hospitals were built and medical education became better organised. The population increased and more people were ill. There were all kinds of new diseases that had not been known before.

The more food was tampered with and altered, the more doctors and hospitals were needed. But these things changed so slowly and so many other aspects of life were transforming that nobody realised what was really happening.

People loved sweet things and wanted more and more of them. Tooth decay became a very common thing, and already by the end of the nineteenth century many dentists were working hard. People started to clean their teeth with toothbrushes.

Nobody was ever satisfied. People had more money and they wanted more food. They wanted food in greater variety, products that came from far-away countries. Businessmen and chemical workers put their heads together and worked out wonderful ideas. There were many problems: the problems of transport, of storage, of keeping the food from spoiling, and there was the problem that when the food became too old, it would lose its taste and colour. Some foods would melt too soon and others would harden. But these clever men found a solution to everything. They added all kinds of chemicals to the food – nice colours, good tastes, substances which kept the food at just the right consistency and, above all, they found chemicals which killed the bacteria in the food so that it could be kept for months and even years. They boiled, bleached and changed food in every possible way. Through all these manipulations and chemicals, the original food, which was meant for the people, has changed completely during the last 60 years – and is still being changed at an ever-increasing speed. But, at the same time, the health of the people is changing more and more and it is hard to find anybody in our Western world who still feels completely healthy and has no complaints.

Chemicals and other additions to our food and all the different manipulations of it were not the only things which altered our lives. Also, the air we breathe, the water we drink and the earth in which our food grows have all changed very much. The smoke of more and more factories pollutes the air. In most cities, the citizens inhale many different chemicals and other waste products every day. By way of the lungs, these chemicals enter the body and all the body cells. The earth in which our food grows and the grass which the animals eat, whose meat we consume, is treated with artificial fertilisers. These fertilisers kill the different fungi and other living organisms which are needed to bring minerals and other essential materials out of the earth into the plants. They are needed as go-between workers, and when they are killed, the plants will grow but they will lack many things and will have less value for our health. Some people even treat the seeds which they sow with different chemicals or certain rays in order to have bigger crops. These treatments guarantee a greater yield, but we do not yet know which valuable parts of the plants might be destroyed in this way and how much the natural cell structure has changed. Aren't we playing with fire?

When the plants grow and the fruit ripens, different kinds of sprays are used. Of course, we have to do this because these sprays are needed to keep away and kill the insects. In nature, on each little piece of land there is always a great variety of plants and trees. In this way, nature is well balanced, everything is in the right proportion and there is no danger that one particular kind of insect will multiply so much that all the plants are destroyed. But if we have big surface areas where only one kind of plant grows, the natural balance is lost, some insects die and others multiply in unnatural numbers. Everywhere that human beings have changed the course of nature, balance is destroyed and problems arise. All the fertilisers and sprays get deep into the earth, into the brooks and streams, into the rivers and into our drinking water. We try to clean this water, but it is very difficult and often new harmful chemicals are found in it. Many of these chemicals get into our body. By way of food alone, each European or American absorbs 2–4 lb (1–2 kg) of pure chemicals each year, and we do not know how much we absorb in other ways. Even if some of those chemicals are not particularly harmful in themselves, the combination of them in our body might be extremely dangerous. Some of these substances are permitted in some countries but strictly forbidden in others. We still know very little about them. Some chemicals dissolve very easily in our body fluids. When these fluids are more or less saturated, there is not much place left for the absorption of all the minerals and other essentials we need. These minerals dissolve with much more difficulty than the chemicals. Our cells lack more and more of the necessary foods, and when they get weak, our health suffers accordingly.

When our cells become weak, they lose their force. Sometimes they lose so much force that they are unable to push their own waste materials out. More and more of these waste products accumulate within the cells until they suffocate completely.

Now, let us take a general look to see what is happening:

- An ever-increasing lack of the necessary building materials weakens our body cells
- More and more harmful substances and chemicals enter our bodies by way of our food, our drinks, the air we inhale and also through our skin
- The quantity of the food we eat is usually far too much. The surplus food which we cannot digest well stays too long in our intestines. This food starts to ferment and rot and many gases and acids result
- When we are tired, sad or overexcited, our food is not digested properly and the same thing happens
- Many medicines bring more chemical toxins into the body and some treatments are so tiring that they take away energy which is badly needed for the process of healing

Now, you already know something about the first two points. The third point is also very important. Most people eat about three to four times the quantity of food that they really need. The first reason for this might be that our modern food is really 'empty', devoid of real, valuable ingredients. In an unconscious way, we try to make up for this lack and eat as much as we can. The second reason is probably our social life. Every gathering, every form of entertainment, every social occasion is centred around eating and drinking. Most things we eat on these occasions are empty calories and nothing else. The third reason may be personal problems, loneliness or boredom. To make up for other things that are missing, we give ourselves the pleasure of eating.

When primitive people stop eating, their intestines are empty within 28 to 34 hours. For people of our Western world, this takes around 72 hours. All this surplus food is slowly spoiling in our digestive channels. If we could see this mixture of all the foods we have eaten during only one day, we would feel completely nauseated. Is it any wonder that we get all kinds of digestive troubles, constipation, diarrhoea and intestinal infections? This incredible food mixture is also a cause of the spoiling of the food within our body, and the enormous amounts of sugar and starches we eat hasten this process. Many gases develop and going to the toilet can be a difficult and painful experience.

Why should we worry? Medical science has made almost unbelievable progress during the last 50 years. There are pills and remedies for every possible ailment. Just take those and your troubles disappear. For your digestion, you take antacids, an aspirin helps many things and, for your headache, there are many different medicines. If one thing does not help you, try another. Eventually, one of them will work. There are remedies for constipation, hundreds of them. For colds, there are syrups, tablets or pills, as many as you can imagine. If you feel bad, you only have to go to the pharmacy and buy something. If a little does not help, you take some more.

If nothing helps and you still feel ill, you go to a doctor and, in nine out of ten cases, the doctor will prescribe other, stronger medicines, the ones which you cannot buy yourself over the counter from the pharmacy. The doctor has to do something about your sickness, they have to give you a prescription, otherwise they would not be a good doctor. We are so completely convinced of this that we do not know any better. Often these medicines help and you feel better. Your symptoms go away and you can go to work. Sometimes you feel a little tired, especially when you have been on antibiotics, but gradually this also passes and you go on living as you used to do, until you become ill again.

If you ever take the time to sit still and think about these things, you will realise that most of the people you know have either slight complaints or are really ill. The more contact you have with people and the more you talk to people, the more you will realise that everyone has at least something the matter with them – and all these people worry about their own health, about the health of their family and the health of their friends, and there are also some people who worry about the health of their countrymen. But only a few of them dare to speak their mind, dare to have the courage to take responsibility for their knowledge. These people realise the looming danger of this general poisoning which goes on in our present modern world. We poison our land, our water and our earth and we poison our own bodies from the outside and also from the inside.

Maybe there are many other people who know what is going on, but they do not dare to use this knowledge. They are very pessimistic, but they do not think that they can do anything about it. But the people who fight against this terrible pollution of the entire earth might be the only people who can still do something about it before it is too late.

People always want to live for today and they do not like to think about future problems, but the time will come when our earth will yield fewer and fewer valuable foods and our water will be completely undrinkable. Then there will be too little oxygen in the air and people will no longer be able to breathe properly. At the same time, they will be completely suffocated by the accumulated poisons in the air. Then life on earth will be impossible for human beings. If we continue at this rate to poison ourselves and our beautiful earth, these times will not be far in the future. Many other races and civilisations have disappeared during the history of our earth, but they were always replaced by new civilisations. This time, it will take a long time before our earth will be habitable again.

All this still seems to be far off and none of our business, but it *is* everybody's business and responsibility. As soon as we realise this great danger, we have to do something about it. And *we can* – if there are only enough people who will wake up from the dream. Knowledge and understanding give people great responsibility.

Never forget that our earth will not be destroyed right away, like the health of primitive people when civilisation comes suddenly. No, most probably this destruction will come bit by bit, and the agony and suffering of millions of people will be indescribable. It has started already, but most people do not seem to realise that this suffering is increasing daily and they think that it has always been like this. They do not see, and they do not want to see, what is happening.

It makes them sad and miserable when people are abnormal, injured, blind, rheumatic or paralysed so that they have to sit in wheelchairs. They look away and forget as fast as they can, and if they can't, they just drink another cocktail. They give something to collections and they donate to certain organisations. This settles their minds and they do not need to think about it any more – they have done their duty. They never look into hidden corners. They do not go to hospitals, clinics or old people's homes where people lie for weeks, months and sometimes even years without any hope of getting better. Sometimes they are in great pain and sometimes only half alive because of the painkillers they get.

What do most people know about children with learning difficulties and all the work and the great sadness they cause their parents? What do they know about all the silent suffering which is going on in so many homes, where members of the family have diabetes, heart troubles, cancer or some other incurable disease? What do they know about all the children who cannot learn at school because they do not get the right nourishment? What do they know about the many unhappy people who cannot live in peace together because they always feel ill and do not have the energy to make an effort to be kind to one another? These people are too listless, too constipated or too weak to keep a happy family together. What a wonderful, happy world this could be . . .

Crime and mental diseases grow at an alarming rate. You may think this has nothing to do with food or with general pollution, but if you already know that the lack of only one vitamin or mineral in our daily food can make people sick, you will understand that young people living solely on soft drinks, ice creams and frankfurters have an immense lack of many essential nutrients. Young people like that cannot be very lovable or well-balanced people. The acids which develop in their bodies from eating this kind of food go into their body fluids and, from there, into every cell of their bodies, including the brain cells. As mentioned earlier in the book, many well-known doctors have come to the conclusion that certain types of mental disease result from food allergies or from a lack of certain minerals. Often these young people start taking drugs and sometimes they do not even realise what they are doing half the time. No, our new generation hasn't got much to smile about. They often do not trust other people, they feel tired, listless and very often unhappy. What is the sense in living like that?

More and more money is being spent – hundreds, thousands and even millions of pounds – and all this money is being used for the building of more and more hospitals, clinics, sanatoriums, old people's homes and so on. It is also used for dental care and medical prevention centres, where people can have a regular check-up or where they can be inoculated against all kinds of diseases. This money pays for hundreds of organisations that help patients who have diabetes, tuberculosis, heart diseases or cancer; and for the building of new universities where more and more students learn about the human body and how to treat people when they are already sick; and the greater part of all this money is spent on research and the development of new medicines.

All these scientists work hard, and each new discovery gives a little gleam of hope that one day we will find something that will prevent all dental decay or even something that will heal cancer. Conscientious doctors often get very little sleep and they give all their attention and time to the constantly growing numbers of patients.

Why, then, do we get the impression that nothing seems to help? That all this work and all this money give so few results? There are always more patients and more diseases. Anyone who looks at statistics covering illness over the last 20 years will be deeply disturbed. The greater part of the population of our Western countries is ill or unable to work because of some chronic or minor disease. Could it be that we are on the wrong track?

Scientists do everything to find the causes of different diseases. They look for microbes, bacteria, viruses and all kinds of other invading micro-organisms, and when they find some that might do harm, they work hard to find a medicine that will destroy them. But if you know something about nature and you have your own little garden, you know that insects never go onto healthy plants. Healthy plants have a great resistance to all kinds of diseases and it seems that they develop a kind of substance, a certain element, which repels the insects that could harm them. Insects only go onto plants that are weak, or onto fruits that are bruised or already beginning to spoil. There they find the environment and the food they like, where they can live and multiply.

With the human body, this also seems to be the case. When a person is strong and healthy, no bacteria or viruses will do them any harm. They might come into the body, but they do not become aggressive. Only when a person is weak, when there is slight imperfection, or when there are toxins and poisons and the body is filled with waste products, will they find the right environment to multiply, and then there will be infections and diseases. They will always look for the weakest part of the body to settle down and make themselves at home.

Now, if we have an infection or any other symptom at a certain weak spot in our body, we will give this symptom a name according to the place where we find it. We talk about ear infections, kidney stones, stomach ulcers and so on, and for each kind of 'disease', as we call them, there are specialists. Most of these diseases are treated as completely different problems which have little or nothing to do with one another. For each of these diseases, there are special medicines that are used to 'heal' them and to suppress the symptoms.

These medicines seem to be a wonderful thing. They make you feel better, your symptoms disappear and you are glad that you are no longer sick. And some other day when you do not feel well again, you will take some aspirin or go to your doctor for the same prescription. If the same medicine does not help you this time, you will ask him for something else, and your troubles will pass. Nobody has time to be ill these days – there is so much work and there are so many social obligations. Whenever you get ill, you want to get rid of the symptoms as fast as possible.

Now, I am *not* telling you *never* to take any medicines. Sometimes the taking of medicines is an absolute necessity. It is then better to take the risk of poisoning yourself a little more rather than suffering intolerable pain or losing your life, or in order to prevent some terrible disease or to heal some serious illness when all natural treatments have failed. When you are well again, if you live sensibly, there will be a good chance that you will be able to expel these poisons again. But never, never, take antibiotics or equally strong chemicals for any minor complaint or give very strong medicines to young children, something which is done far too often. You might ruin their health and the health of many future generations in that way. Human life is far too precious and living can be so wonderful.

But what really does happen when you take medicines and your troubles disappear? As I said earlier, symptoms of 'disease' are signs that the body is attempting to eliminate toxins. Maybe you have a temperature, by which some of these waste products are destroyed. But then, in the midst of this cleansing process, you interfere and this work cannot be continued. Your body temperature becomes normal again and no more toxins can be destroyed. No further toxins can leave your body. They are suppressed by the medicine you have taken, and as they cannot leave, they go back to where they came from, and they go even deeper into the body. As some of the toxins have had an opportunity to leave your body before you took the medicine, the number of them that goes deeper into your body is a little less than before. But added to these are the new toxins from the medicine you have taken. Everything which is not part of the body, or is not of the same intrinsic construction as the body cells, is harmful to the body. But now you are happy because you feel better, and you do not worry about toxins you do not notice. But slowly, through your food and several other causes, new harmful substances are added to the old ones and pressure builds up again. After some time, a new explosion follows and this is considered a new disease and is treated by another specialist with another kind of medicine. And so a vicious circle starts, and you and your doctor probably never realise that all these different troubles have one and the same cause – the saturation of your entire body with substances which are harmful and should not be there.

When people are young, when their bodies still have plenty of energy in storage for their defence, the reactions against the saturation of their body fluids will be strong. These kind of reactions are called 'acute' illnesses. These are like sudden explosions. But when people get older and lose much of their strength, these reactions become weaker but they repeat themselves more often. These are called 'chronic' diseases. Especially when suffering from these kinds of diseases, people go on taking the same kind of medicines over a long period. As a result, their body fluids become more and more saturated and, at the same time, their body cells become weaker and weaker.

Many people have been eating the almost empty foods of our 'civilised' countries for many years. This food is lacking almost entirely in the most important minerals and other building materials which we need and it contains many harmful substances. At the same time, these people may have some chronic minor or more serious disease for which they always take some kind of medicine. Often these people work very hard, without taking a real holiday or time off to relax, and if they also have many worries or personal problems which are getting them down, their body will not be able to fight any more. All body fluids and body cells will be completely saturated with waste materials and will slowly be poisoned from within. Their cells will become very weak and will contain less and less oxygen.

This is the last stage, when nothing functions normally any more. Their chronic disease might become very serious. They may get a heart attack or a serious form of diabetes, and maybe their body cells will go mad and not obey any natural law any more. These cells will start multiplying and multiplying and these people will have 'cancer'. This is the end of the line, the last stage of an endless intoxication which has been building up over many, many years. This cancer will always start at the weakest part of the body, where it finds the least resistance. There it can slowly develop, until some day this person will realise that they are a victim of this terrible disease.

Huge sums of money are spent daily on cancer research. Hundreds of scientists try to find a bacterium, a virus or another micro-organism that could be the cause of cancer. There has to be a scapegoat. More and more carcinogenic substances are discovered and these are mostly food or products which we use daily. When people have spent thousands more pounds, one day they will discover that *every food* and *every product* which is not completely natural and contains substances other than it should contain by its natural law is carcinogenic. None of these products is the original cause of cancer; they are only the last drop of poison as a result of which the poison bucket flows over.

When all your cells are filled with waste products, and all your body fluids are saturated with toxins, there is only one very tiny bit of poison needed to start a chain reaction which will cause cells to begin to multiply.

Some doctors say that cancer is a 'mental process' – a problem of the mind. There is much truth in this statement. If you are not happy, your digestion is bad and your entire body works with much less efficiency. In the same way, you can poison your body by a steady accumulation of waste materials. Happy and optimistic people have a far better chance of staying healthy and less chance of getting cancer. I do not mean noisy and nervous people – they also have a bad digestion and many troubles. I mean people who are really happy and well balanced. A happy disposition is the greatest defence against disease, but when we absorb many toxins, our health declines and we lose our gaiety and our natural confidence.

The more we think about all these problems, the more pessimistic we become. It seems that there is no hope and no way out of all this misery for the human race. We are poisoned and threatened from every possible side and even from within our own bodies – by the air, the water and the earth, and most of all by our fellow human beings who close their eyes and do not see, or do not want to see, what is happening. They do not seem to realise that if they destroy all living things on our beautiful earth, they themselves, their children and all future generations will also be destroyed.

This chapter might appear to be all gloom and doom, but it is not as bad as all that. There is always sunshine behind the clouds, and in a world full of problems, good health can still be achieved. It may seem that the threats to our health, happiness and vitality are overwhelming, but we should not be without hope. We all have the ability to make choices and take action, for our own good and that of our world.

CHAPTER THIRTEEN

Conclusion

No one should ever make accusations or critical observations without at least trying to give a solution to the problems mentioned. I believe absolutely in the intrinsic goodness and the longing for health and happiness in every human being. Many people who seem bad or disagreeable are simply the victims of their education, their surroundings, the strain of modern life and, most of all, their own failing health. But at the end of the day, every human being of every race and colour has the same kind of dream about a happy life and a better future.

Bad behaviour, disagreements and opposition to all new ideas are often the consequences of a lack of knowledge and understanding, and a fear of the unknown. When you approach a human being from the right angle, in the right way, they will always be friendly and cooperative. It is the same with animals. If you aren't afraid and if you are friendly to a dog, it will wag its tail, but if you are frightened, it will growl and bark and possibly even bite you. If people really understood how much they could help themselves and the people they love by learning a bit more about becoming, being and staying healthy, each one of them would do his utmost to help.

One person can do a little, many people can do more and millions of people can change the world. The most important thing is education – health education of the masses. When they become more knowledgeable about food and what is good for them, all these millions of people will demand better and healthier food, and fewer toxins and poisons in their environment.

I am no fanatic. I enjoy living and, once in a while, I even enjoy eating the forbidden fruit. If a person is healthy, they can, now and again, eat or drink something that is *not* very healthy. Our body is a wonderful gift and it contains a strong vital force for its defence. We can permit ourselves to be tempted from time to time. These poisons will be excreted if you pay a little more attention to the things you eat after going on a spree like that, but it is an entirely different thing if our daily intake of food contains only calories and little else.

Nobody should change their eating habits overnight. Nothing should ever be forced. If, all of a sudden, we were again to start eating the food of our forefathers, like raw fish and raw meat, some insects, bird eggs, oil, fruits, berries, herbs, nuts and a few soft bones, most of us would become ill and nothing would be gained.

It is very regrettable that some people who have been seriously ill at some time in their lives and who have recovered thanks to some special natural diet are convinced that all other people will be able to recover, to be healthy and to stay healthy by eating exactly the same kind of diet. More than one road leads to Rome!

Through the ages, while people have been eating many different kinds of food, our digestive juices have changed and also our saliva has a slightly different composition now. Taste and smell have declined. What is good for one person is not necessarily good for another, and although somebody might gain great benefits from following a certain diet, this diet may even be harmful to another person. Each one of us lacks different minerals, vitamins or other nutrients, and because of this, our bodies need different kinds of food. Raw vegetables or fruits are very healthy, but some people cannot digest them and have to become accustomed to them very slowly.

For this reason, there is so much misunderstanding about natural health and all kinds of diets. Of course everybody should become familiar with the right food again – the food we really need – but in nature it is not possible to make sudden changes. Very carefully, our digestive systems will have to become reaccustomed to the absorption and the use of natural food. Eventually, everybody will get used to this kind of food again, and then the health of the entire population of our Western world will improve.

In other ways, too, sudden changes can often do more harm than good. We cannot say that, from now on, we will do away with doctors and medicine, factories that make food preservatives, or modern agriculture with its use of sprays or fertilisers. In such cases, what we need is to carefully adapt to better ways.

We will always need doctors. We will have accidents, operations will have to be performed and there will always be sick people who need care. But the role the doctor plays in our lives will have to be changed. Medical students learn many valuable things. Their working programme is already overloaded, but they learn very little about the original cause of all diseases and how to treat them according to the laws of nature. They are taught nothing about the important role our daily food plays as the cause and also as the healing factor in most of our diseases, nor do they know that nature is our greatest healing force. Have they really forgotten that Hippocrates did not like the use of strong medicines and told us to watch nature as the best example?

All wild animals are far healthier than human beings. When an animal is hurt or feels ill, it lies down in a quiet corner, stops eating and only drinks a little water until it feels well again. If all of us had the courage to do the same thing, there would be many more healthy people and fewer diseases. In natural medicine, we use the following method which is the most valuable one: we rest and we eat nothing or only a small amount of light food until our problems have passed, and afterwards we will be even healthier than before.

As I have said, the role of the doctor has to be revised. We need doctors, maybe more than ever, but their work should mainly be the work of a teacher. They should teach us what to do when we are sick and not just take out a pen and write a prescription. They have to make people understand how their bodies work and how they can keep their bodies healthy and strong. Only where there is real need, in order to give help in cases of unbearable pain or suffering, should doctors make use of their knowledge about modern remedies and treatments.

We should not abolish *all* medicines, but we should keep in mind the words spoken some time ago at an international convention of the World Health Organisation in Geneva: 'There are some 2,000 different medicines but, in reality, we only need about 150 of them to treat all existing diseases.'

We still need our food factories, but there are better and more natural ways of food preservation, food colouring and other procedures. Factories will always produce what the public demands and they will always be in business. When factory owners start to understand why so many people are ill, they will cooperate, and not only their customers but also their own families and friends will become healthier. Gradually, they will also change their packing material to more natural versions. They will buy more natural and unspoilt foods. Because of this change in demand, agriculture will also slowly change. More and more natural food will be grown and it will be cultivated on smaller plots of land. The earth will have the opportunity to rebuild its natural composition and its balance. Fewer and fewer insects will destroy the harvest.

Conclusion

One thing leads to another. Slowly but surely, things can be changed. When the first step has been taken, then others will follow and step by step we will climb up the ladder again from which we have been falling down with ever-increasing speed during the last 100 years, and especially during the last 20 or 30 years. The only thing we need is the complete cooperation of every man, woman and child as soon as they understand the danger. Everyone should demand healthier and better food. Let us get organised and let the people with courage and understanding lead the way. If we do not do this, we will fall down the ladder of health at increasing speed until the total destruction of health is complete and there only remains a slow and terrible death for all human beings.

So what is the answer? Health and vitality is a convergence of minds. Mind is stronger than body. If we put ourselves in a positive frame of mind, in the short time we are here on this earth we can lead a healthy, happy life, full of vitality. We just need to make a few changes so that our body can reap the rewards. It is amazing how much our body is capable of doing for us. If, for instance, we have a small cut, we can see the healing process start. With a little effort on our part, we can achieve a great deal. All this is worthwhile if we want to lead more fulfilling lives. Remember that, for the little while we are here on this earth, if we really want to enjoy life with a vision of happiness, then we need to put our minds to it.

Index